# Methods in Molecular Biology

*Series Editor*
John M. Walker
School of Life Sciences
University of Hertfordshire
Hatfield, Hertfordshire, AL10 9AB, UK

For further volumes:
http://www.springer.com/series/7651

# T-Helper Cells

## Methods and Protocols

Edited by

**Ari Waisman**

*Institute for Molecular Medicine, University Medical Center of the Johannes Gutenberg University of Mainz, Mainz, Germany*

**Burkhard Becher**

*Institute of Experimental Immunology, University of Zurich, Zurich, Germany*

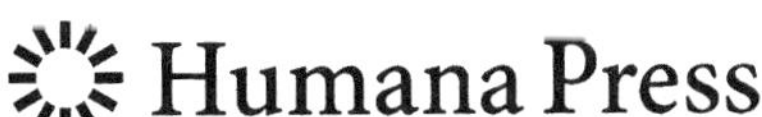

*Editors*
Ari Waisman
Institute for Molecular Medicine
University Medical Center of the
Johannes Gutenberg University of Mainz
Mainz, Germany

Burkhard Becher
Institute of Experimental Immunology
University of Zurich
Zurich, Germany

ISSN 1064-3745 ISSN 1940-6029 (electronic)
ISBN 978-1-4939-1211-7 ISBN 978-1-4939-1212-4 (eBook)
DOI 10.1007/978-1-4939-1212-4
Springer New York Heidelberg Dordrecht London

Library of Congress Control Number: 2014945206



Printed on acid-free paper

Humana Press is a brand of Springer
Springer is part of Springer Science+Business Media (www.springer.com)

## Preface

Ever since the discovery of "cellular antibodies" in the 1960s [1] it became evident that adaptive immune responses are dependent on antibody-producing B cells and thymus-derived T cells [2]. After the T cell receptors of mice and men were cloned [3, 4], it became clear that T cells mastermind cellular and humoral immune responses. In particular $CD4^+$ T helper ($T_H$) cells are critical for the development of immunological memory and immune regulation.

$T_H$ cells were later subdivided into $T_H1$ and $T_H2$ cells based on their ability to produce distinct sets of cytokines [5] and therefore to specifically mediate different immune responses to cellular vs. extracellular threats. An additional subset of regulatory/suppressor $T_H$ cells was postulated already in the 1970 [6], but only with the discovery of FoxP3 as a critical transcription factor for their development were Tregs accepted as a unique and independent member of the growing family of $T_H$ cell subsets [7–9]. Apart perhaps from Tregs, there appears to be a large degree of plasticity in terms of functional and phenotypic specialization amongst $T_H$ cells. Other subsets, such as TGFβ-secreting $T_H3$ cells, $T_H17$ cells (IL-17 producing), $T_H9$ cells (IL-9 producing), and $T_H22$ cells (IL-22 producing), have led to the erroneous assumption that such polarization patterns are hardwired and irreversible. Instead, it has become clear that these new T cell subsets are rarely found in vivo (at least in mice) and that their polarization is vastly plastic and reversible.

To capture the unique features of $T_H$ cells, which are critical for host defense, but must also be blamed for numerous chronic inflammatory diseases, novel tools had to be developed for the isolation of $T_H$ cells from various tissues and subsequent analysis of their functional properties in vitro, ex vivo, and in vivo. Here, we have invited specialists in $T_H$ cell biology to share their most efficient and current protocols for the study of this amazingly versatile and potent cell type.

In this book, we have put together a few "recipes" focusing on working with T cells of mice and men. In the first four chapters, von *Stebut*, *Greter*, *Hövelmeyer*, *Kurts*, and colleagues describe methods of isolating T cells from various tissues in mice, which permit the characterization and in vitro culture of these cells immediately ex vivo. The next five chapters by *Mair*, *Tosevski*, *Newell*, *Ruland*, *Sparwasser*, and their colleagues are dedicated to protocols for the analysis of T cell function and phenotype using various cutting-edge technologies. The next three chapters by *Zielinski*, *Segal*, *Fillatreau*, and colleagues describe methods allowing for the manipulation of T cell function in vitro and in vivo. The final seven chapters by *Taube*, *Weigmann*, *Buch*, *Clausen*, *Anderton*, *Maloy*, *Heikenwälder*, and their colleagues are dedicated to in vivo models of diseases in which T cells play a central role in the pathogenesis.

This is not an all-encompassing compendium of all the available tools and technologies to study T cells, but a relatively broad selection of cutting-edge protocols to enable the reader to immediately apply them at the bench. If a specific subject is missing, we are confident that the creative lab scientist will be able to adapt the protocol to suit his/her needs and to add the newly developed protocol to this ever-growing list of methods to study this fascinating leukocyte, the helper T cell.

*Zürich, Switzerland* *Burkhard Becher*
*Mainz, Germany* *Ari Waisman*

## References


1. Govaerts A (1960) Cellular antibodies in kidney homotransplantation. J Immunol 85: 516–522
2. Miller JF, Mitchell GF (1967) The thymus and the precursors of antigen reactive cells. Nature 216:659–663
3. Yanagi Y, Yoshikai Y, Leggett K, Clark SP, Aleksander I, Mak TW (1984) A human T cell-specific cDNA clone encodes a protein having extensive homology to immunoglobulin chains. Nature 308:145–9
4. Hedrick SM, Cohen DI, Nielsen EA, Davis MM (1984) Isolation of cDNA clones encoding T cell-specific membrane-associated proteins. Nature 308:149–53
5. Mosmann TR, Coffman RL (1989) TH1 and TH2 cells: different patterns of lymphokine secretion lead to different functional properties. Annu Rev Immunol 7: 145–173
6. Gershon RK, Kondo K (1970) Cell interactions in the induction of tolerance: the role of thymic lymphocytes. Immunology 18:723–737
7. Fontenot JD, Gavin MA, Rudensky AY (2003) Foxp3 programs the development and function of CD4+CD25+ regulatory T cells. Nat Immunol 4:330–336
8. Hori S, Nomura T, Sakaguchi S (2003) Control of regulatory T cell development by the transcription factor Foxp3. Science 299: 1057–1061
9. Khattri R, Cox T, Yasayko SA, Ramsdell F (2003) An essential role for Scurfin in CD4+CD25+ T regulatory cells. Nat Immunol 4:337–342

# Contents

## Contributors


STEPHEN M. ANDERTON • *MRC Centre for Inflammation Research and Centre for Multiple Sclerosis Research, Queen's Medical Research Institute, University of Edinburgh, Edinburgh, UK*

BURKHARD BECHER • *Institute of Experimental Immunology, University of Zürich, Zürich, Switzerland*

JULIA M. BRAUN • *Cellular Immunoregulation, Department of Dermatology and Allergology, Charité-Universitätsmedizin, Berlin, Germany*

THORSTEN BUCH • *Institute for Medical Microbiology, Immunology and Hygiene, Technische Universität München, Munich, Germany*

HELEN E. CAMBROOK • *MRC Centre for Inflammation Research and Centre for Multiple Sclerosis Research, Queen's Medical Research Institute, University of Edinburgh, Edinburgh, UK*

B.E. CLAUSEN • *Institute for Molecular Medicine, University Medical Center, Johannes Gutenberg-University, Mainz, Germany*

LYNSEY FAIRBAIRN • *Institute for Medical Microbiology, Immunology and Hygiene, Technische Universität München, Munich, Germany*

SIMON FILLATREAU • *Deutsches Rheuma-ForschungsZentrum, a Leibniz Institute, Berlin, Germany*

OLIVER GORKA • *Institut für Klinische Chemie und Pathobiochemie, Klinikum rechts der Isar, Technische Universität München, Munich, Germany*

MELANIE GRETER • *Institute of Experimental Immunology, University of Zürich, Zürich, Switzerland*

CHRISTOPHER HACKENBRUCH • *Institute for Molecular Medicine, University Medical Center, Johannes Gutenberg-University, Mainz, Germany*

MATHIAS HEIKENWÄLDER • *Institute of Virology, Technische Universität München, Helmholtz Zentrum München für Gesundheit und Umwelt (HMGU), Munich, Germany*

ELLEN HILGENBERG • *Deutsches Rheuma-ForschungsZentrum, a Leibniz Institute, Berlin, Germany*

NADINE HÖVELMEYER • *Institute for Molecular Medicine, University Medical Center, Johannes Gutenberg-University, Mainz, Germany*

ELISA KIEBACK • *Max Delbrueck Center for Molecular Medicine, Berlin, Germany*

CHRISTIAN KURTS • *Institute of Experimental Immunology, University of Bonn, Bonn, Germany*

IVA LELIOS • *Institute of Experimental Immunology, University of Zürich, Zürich, Switzerland*

BEATE LORENZ • *Department of Dermatology, University Medical Center, Johannes Gutenberg University, Mainz, Germany*

ISIS LUDWIG-PORTUGALL • *Institute of Experimental Immunology, Rheinische Friedrich-Wilhelms-University of Bonn, Bonn, Germany*

FLORIAN MAIR • *Institute of Experimental Immunology, University of Zürich, Zürich, Switzerland*

KEVIN J. MALOY • *Sir William Dunn School of Pathology, University of Oxford, Oxford, UK*

CHRISTIAN THOMAS MAYER • *Institute of Infection Immunology, TWINCORE/Centre for Experimental and Clinical Infection Research; a joint venture between the Medical School Hannover (MHH) and the Helmholtz Centre for Infection Research (HZI), Hannover, Germany*

RHOANNE C. MCPHERSON • *MRC Centre for Inflammation Research and Centre for Multiple Sclerosis Research, Queen's Medical Research Institute, University of Edinburgh, Edinburgh, UK*

HELEN MEYER-MARTIN • *Department of Medicine, University Medical Center, Mainz, Germany*

EVAN W. NEWELL • *Singapore Immunology Network (SIgN), Agency for Science Technology and Research (A-STAR), Singapore, Singapore*

RICHARD A. O'CONNOR • *MRC Centre for Inflammation Research and Centre for Multiple Sclerosis Research, Queen's Medical Research Institute, University of Edinburgh, Edinburgh, UK*

J.L. OBER-BLÖBAUM • *Institute for Molecular Medicine, University Medical Center, Johannes Gutenberg-University, Mainz, Germany*

S. PANTELYUSHIN • *Institute of Experimental Immunology, University of Zürich, Zürich, Switzerland*

SONJA REIßIG • *Institute for Molecular Medicine, University Medical Center, Johannes Gutenberg-University, Mainz, Germany*

SEBASTIAN REUTER • *Department of Medicine, University Medical Center, Mainz, Germany*

JÜRGEN RULAND • *Institut für Klinische Chemie und Pathobiochemie, Klinikum rechts der Isar, Technische Universität München, Munich, Germany*

JULIE RUMBLE • *Holtom-Garrett Program in Neuroimmunology and Multiple Sclerosis Center, Department of Neurology, University of Michigan, Ann Arbor, MI, USA*

BENJAMIN M. SEGAL • *Holtom-Garrett Program in Neuroimmunology and Multiple Sclerosis Center, Department of Neurology, University of Michigan, Ann Arbor, MI, USA*

ANNA ŚLEDZIŃSKA • *Institute of Experimental Immunology, University of Zürich, Zürich, Switzerland*

GEORGE X. SONG-ZHAO • *Sir William Dunn School of Pathology, University of Oxford, Oxford, UK*

TIM SPARWASSER • *Institute of Infection Immunology, TWINCORE/Centre for Experimental and Clinical Infection Research; a joint venture between the Medical School Hannover (MHH) and the Helmholtz Centre for Infection Research (HZI), Hannover, Germany*

CHRISTIAN TAUBE • *Department of Pneumology, Leiden University Medical Center, Leiden, The Netherlands*

VINKO TOSEVSKI • *Institute of Experimental Immunology, University of Zürich, Zürich, Switzerland*

KRISTIAN UNGER • *Research Unit of Radiation Cytogenetics, Helmholtz-Zentrum München für Gesundheit und Umwelt (HMGU), Neuherberg, Germany*

ESTHER VON STEBUT • *Department of Dermatology, University Medical Center, Johannes Gutenberg University, Mainz, Germany*

ARI WAISMAN • *Institute for Molecular Medicine, University Medical Center of the Johannes Gutenberg University of Mainz, Mainz, Germany*

STEFAN WANNINGER • *Institut für Klinische Chemie und Pathobiochemie, Klinikum rechts der Isar, Technische Universität München, Munich, Germany*
BENNO WEIGMANN • *Medical Clinic, Research-Campus, University of Erlangen-Nuremberg, Erlangen, Germany*
C.T. WOHN • *Erasmus MC, Department of Immunology, University Medical Center Rotterdam, GE Rotterdam, The Netherlands*
LAI LI YUN • *Singapore Immunology Network (SIgN), Agency for Science Technology and Research (A-STAR), Singapore, Singapore*
CHRISTINA E. ZIELINSKI • *Cellular Immunoregulation, Department of Dermatology and Allergology, Charité-Universitätsmedizin Berlin and Berlin-Brandenburg Center for Regenerative Therapies, Charité-Universitätsmedizin, Berlin, Germany; AG Zelluläre Immunregulation, Klinik für Dermatologie und Allergologie, Charité-Universitätsmedizin Berlin, Berlin, Germany*

# Part I

## Isolation of T Cells from the Tissues

# Chapter 1

# Isolation of T Cells from the Skin


## Beate Lorenz and Esther von Stebut



## Abstract

T cells can be found in skin under steady-state conditions as well as in inflammatory processes. T cells in skin play an important role in immune homeostasis as well as control of infectious, inflammatory diseases or tumors. In addition, several important and frequent skin diseases such as psoriasis, atopic dermatitis, autoimmune disease, and contact allergy are initiated by T cells. In skin diseases, the majority of antigen-specific T cells can be found in the tissue, not the peripheral blood. Here, we present a protocol suitable for isolation of skin-resident (inflammatory) T cells that can be used for an in-depth characterization of their frequency, function, and role for the respective inflammatory condition.



**Key words** Skin, T cells, Inflammation


## 1 Introduction

T cells are present in normal human skin in low numbers; upon inflammation, they are strongly recruited to the skin to contribute to resulting immunity. Interestingly, nearly twice as many T cells are present in skin as compared to the circulation [1].

Under steady-state conditions, the main function of cutaneous T cells appears to be immunosurveillance [2]. This is supported by the fact that transplant recipients receiving T cell immunosuppression have a greatly increased risk of developing skin tumors [3]. In addition, skin-resident T cells have been implicated in the development of psoriasis. T cells resident in nonlesional skin from psoriatic patients can divide and induce spontaneous psoriasis lesions upon transplantation of skin onto immunodeficient mice [4]. T cells resident in normal skin can therefore contribute actively to inflammatory skin disease in addition to providing immunosurveillance.

A large number of skin diseases are known to be initiated or controlled by T cells [5, 6]. As such, a strong immigration of T cells into skin during disease development is observed. Here, in the context of T cell-initiated processes, autoimmune diseases such as psoriasis [7, 8], autoimmune blistering diseases, connective


Ari Waisman and Burkhard Becher (eds.), *T-Helper Cells: Methods and Protocols*, Methods in Molecular Biology, vol. 1193, DOI 10.1007/978-1-4939-1212-4_1,

tissue diseases, graft-versus-host disease, and cutaneous allergic inflammation [9] are induced by aberrant T cells. In addition, control and healing of several infectious diseases (e.g., infections with *Mycobacteria*, *Leishmania* [15], etc.) and other conditions such as wound healing [10] and antitumor responses depend on the initiation of antigen-specific T cells against the relevant structures.

Many prior studies have used peripheral blood lymphocytes or—in experimental models—T cells isolated from spleens or lymph nodes to study skin-specific T cell responses. Due to the fact that tissue-homing T cells exhibit a higher antigen-specific frequency and the notion that peripheral blood T cells often do not reflect the local situation with regard to, e.g., Th subset distribution in the respective inflammation [11], the results of such studies are of limited relevance. Interestingly, priming through skin-derived dendritic cells (DC) leads to preferential induction of skin-homing T cells via CCR4 [12], whereas priming through, e.g., the gut to induction of gut-specific T cell subsets.

Thus, to assess the specific role of T cells and their subsets for skin disease onset, regulation and control, isolation, quantification, and characterization of T cells in skin are required. Here, we present a protocol suitable for an in-depth characterization of inflammatory infiltrates in skin [13]. As such, T cells invading the skin due to local triggers can be assessed in detail using surface marker characterization, intracellular FACS staining, or else. Finally, if desired, skin T cells can be enriched from the isolated inflammatory cells using flow cytometric sorting and/or microbeads. This protocol combining enzymatic digestion with mechanical disruption has several advantages: (1) isolation of primary skin cells ex vivo; (2) the procedure is simple and quick; (3) the cell yields are high enough to warrant further applications; and (4) the phenotype of the resulting cells is well characterized; viability of T cells is good [13]. A large number of studies have used the abovementioned or related protocols for high-quality research [13–16].

## 2 Materials

Medium and all working solutions are stored at 4 °C.

### 2.1 Mice

All strains of mice are suitable. However, the majority of our experience was obtained with C57BL/6 or BALB/c inbred strains. Make sure to use lineage markers for cell characterization that are suitable for each specific mouse strain.

### 2.2 Solutions

1. RPMI complete medium (1×): Use RPMI 1640 and add 5 % FCS, 1 % Pen Strep, 1 % nonessential amino acids (NEA, 100× concentrate, Biochrom, Berlin, Germany), 10 mM HEPES buffer, 2 mM L-glutamine, 0.05 mM 2-mercaptoethanol. Sterilize by filtration and store at 4 °C.

2. Phosphate-buffered saline (PBS; 1×): Dissolve 16.08 g NaCl and 2.76 g $NaH_2PO_4 \cdot 1\ H_2O$ in aqua dest. and add volume up to 2 L. Adjust pH to 7.3. Autoclave, store at 4 °C, and prepare with 5 % fetal bovine serum.
3. Enzymatic medium: RPMI medium containing 0.4 mg/mL liberase (Roche) and penicillin/streptavidin; prepare freshly each time.
4. Anti-mouse CD4 (L3T4) MicroBeads, anti-mouse CD8a (Ly-2) MicroBeads.
5. Gentle MACS (Octo) dissociator with Gentle MACS C tubes (all Miltenyi), alternatively: Medimachine, Medicon 50 μm (all Becton Dickinson).
6. 14-Gauge needle and syringe (Becton Dickinson), 6-well plates, cell strainers (70 μm mesh sizes), sterile scissors, incubator (37 °C, 5 % $CO_2$), centrifuge.

## 3 Methods

Perform all procedures at room temperature and sterile conditions; if needed using a laminar flow.

### *3.1 Harvesting of Inflamed Skin, Enzymatic Digestion*

The optimal time point for harvesting inflammatory cells from skin may vary from model to model and needs to be optimized. Generally, cell numbers are highest at the time of maximum skin infiltration noticed by edema and erythema (*see* **Note 1**).

1. Inflamed skin is excised, soaked in 70 % ethanol, and washed with PBS.
2. Tissue samples as large as one ear can be used; if larger, cut in pieces and separate. Ears are split into halves, and cartilage is removed.
3. Skin pieces are deposited in 1.5 mL liberase medium per 6-well and incubated for 1.5 h at 37 °C (5 % $CO_2$).
4. Add 1.5 mL RPMI complete medium per 6-well for inactivation.

### *3.2 Mechanical Isolation of Inflammatory Cells from Skin*

For utilization of a Gentle MACS (*see* **Note 2**):

1. Transfer both halves of one ear (or equal amounts of skin pieces) into a Gentle MACS C Tube containing 1 mL RPMI complete medium.
2. Tightly close the C Tube and attach it upside down onto the sleeve of the Gentle MACS Dissociator. Run the Gentle MACS Program C.
3. Once the program is finished, detach C Tube from the Gentle MACS Dissociator.

Alternatively, the protocol can also be used for cell isolation with a Medimachine:

1A. Transfer skin into green Medicon (50 μm), and remove lid beforehand.

2A. Add 1 mL RPMI medium, close, and run Medimachine for 7 min.

3A. Rinse Medicon with 10 mL RPMI complete medium, gently turn scissors in Medicon with hands, and rinse again with 10 mL of RPMI complete medium.

4. Apply cell solutions from **steps 1** to **3** or **1A** to **3A** to a cell strainer (70 μm mesh size) placed on a 50 mL tube.
5. Discard cell strainer and centrifuge sample at $200 \times g$ for 8 min.
6. Resuspend pellet in PBS, and count cells (*see* **Note 3**, Fig. 1). For one ear, expect to isolate ~$1–2 \times 10^6$ cells per ear under steady-state conditions, up to ×10-fold more in inflammations.

### 3.3 Further Studies Using Skin Inflammatory Cells

#### 3.3.1 Composition of Cellular Infiltrate, Characterization of T Cells

In a next step, depending on the inflammatory nature of the disease state investigated, the composition of the inflammatory skin infiltrate can be analyzed.

As shown in Fig. 2, not all inflammatory conditions of skin lead to T cell immigration. As described, benzalkonium chloride (BAC) leads to a strong skin irritation with edema; however, the inflammatory cells mainly consist of neutrophils. Even at the peak of the infiltration with highest ear swelling responses, hardly any T cells can be identified in the infiltrates. This underlines the specificity of the method described here. In contrast, re-challenge of sensitized mouse ears with the contact allergen TNCB leads to recruitment of up to 7 % of $CD4^+$ T cells into skin (*see* **Note 4**). Using flow cytometry, these infiltrating T cells can next be subdivided into different Th subsets using various markers.

Cutaneous leishmaniasis is a protozoan skin infection, which is ultimately healed in a T cell-dependent manner. IFNγ production by $CD4^+$ Th1 and $CD8^+$ Tc1 cells leads to lesion resolution. As shown in Fig. 3, infection with $10^3$ parasites leads to a strong immigration of T cells into the skin over the course of several weeks. In our hands, mechanical disruption of the skin with the Gentle MACS device provided better T cell yields as compared to the Medimachine. Interestingly, enzymatic digestion did not hamper T cell identification using the markers depicted. The numbers of T cells isolated from a mouse ear at the indicated time points are depicted in Figs. 4 and 5; it can be up to $3 \times 10^6$ for $CD4^+$ T cells and up to $1 \times 10^6$ for $CD8^+$ T cells (*see* **Note 5**).

#### 3.3.2 Isolation of T Cells from Inflammatory Cells

Isolation of T cells from suspensions of skin inflammatory cells is possible (Table 1). These cells can then be used for additional applications such as in-depth analyses of T cell-specific features and adoptive transfers into other host mice.

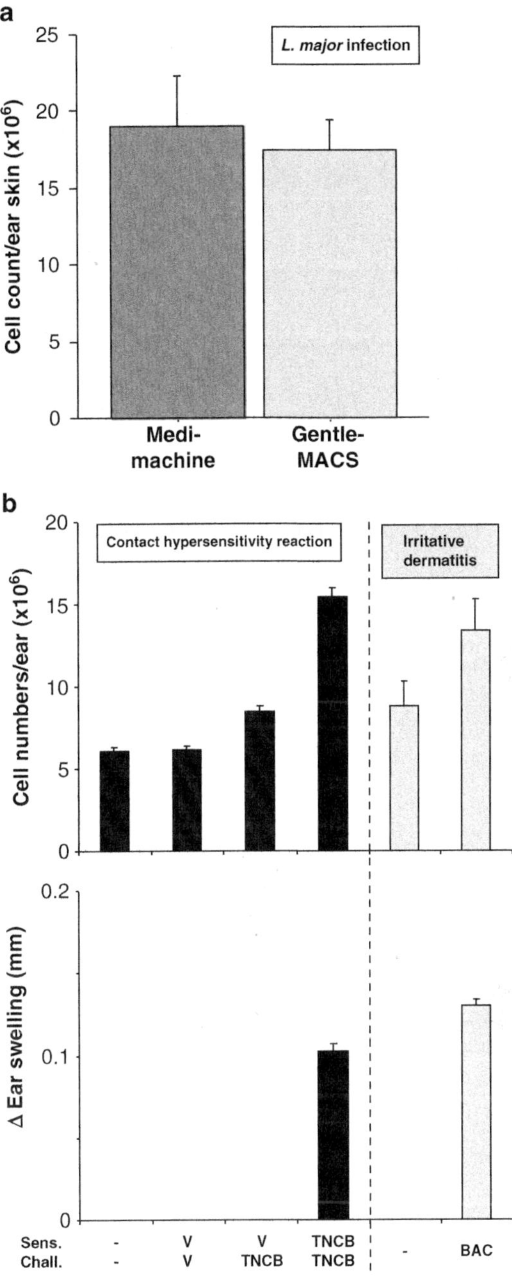


**Fig. 1** Inflammatory cell numbers harvested from ear skin. (**a**) Mice were infected with $2 \times 10^5$ *L. major* parasites. In week 6, ears were harvested and cells isolated as described in this protocol. Cell numbers were determined after cell isolation using different devices ($n = 4$–5 mice/device). (**b**) C57BL/6 mice were sensitized/treated with 450 μg TNCB or 5 % benzalkonium chloride (BAC). In contact hypersensitivity reactions (CHS), 1:3 olive oil/acetone was included as vehicle control (V). Five days later, ears were challenged with 45 μg TNCB. In both CHS- and BAC-induced irritation, ear swelling was assessed after 24 h using a caliper. Ears were harvested and inflammatory cells isolated as described. All data are shown as mean ± SEM, $n = 9$ independent experiments with 26 mice/group for CHS, $n = 4$ independent experiments with 12 mice/group

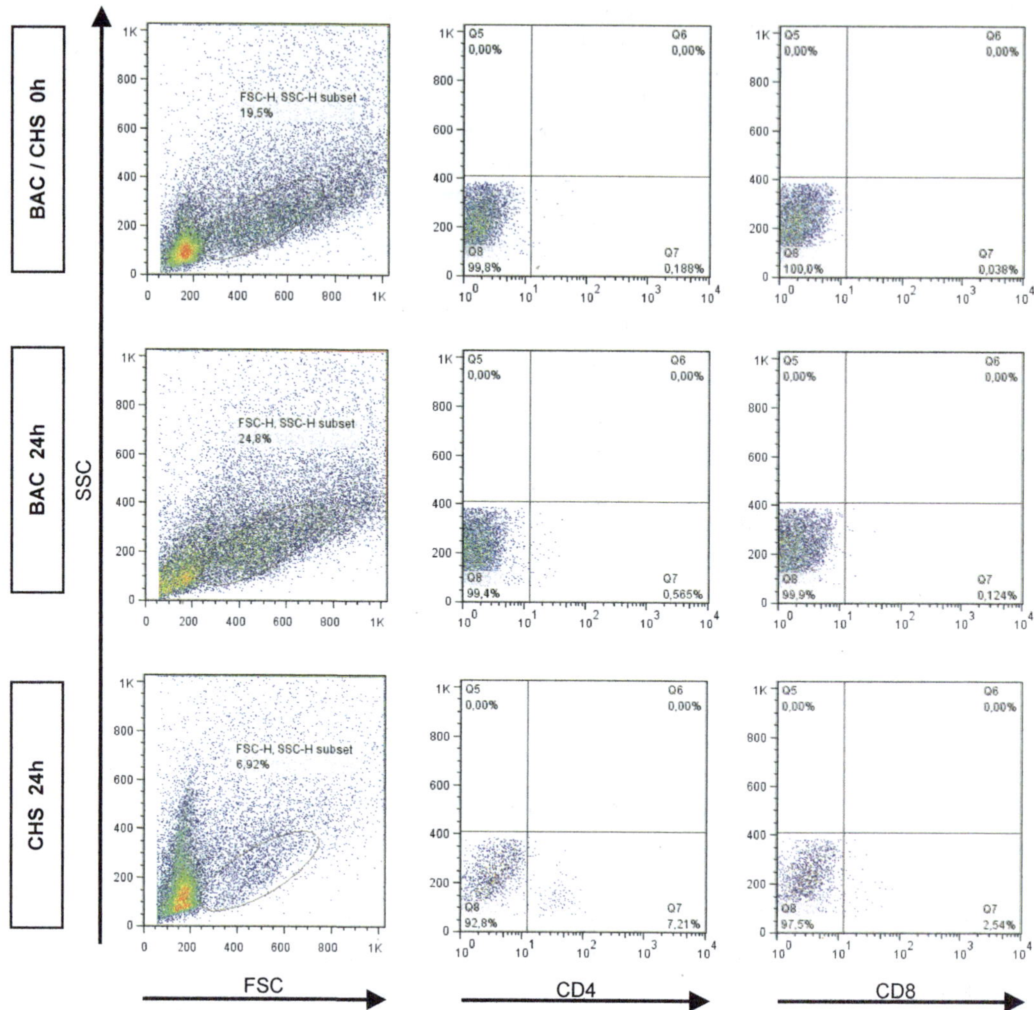


**Fig. 2** Flow cytometric detection of T cells in inflammatory cell suspensions. CHS and irritative contact dermatitis against BAC were initiated as described in Fig. 1. After 24 h, isolated cells were stained with anti-CD4 and anti-CD8 to determine T cell frequencies. Representative FACS stainings are depicted

1. Expect up to ~5 % of your cells to be T cells ($CD3^+$, $CD4^+$, $CD8^+$) in the inflammatory cell suspensions. This may depend on the nature of the condition as well.
2. Use anti-CD4 or anti-CD8 microbeads and the manufacturer's instructions for isolation procedures. Alternatively, flow cytometric cell sorting has been used with good success allowing for a preselection of several key T cell markers (activation markers, markers for regulatory T cells, etc.) at the same time.

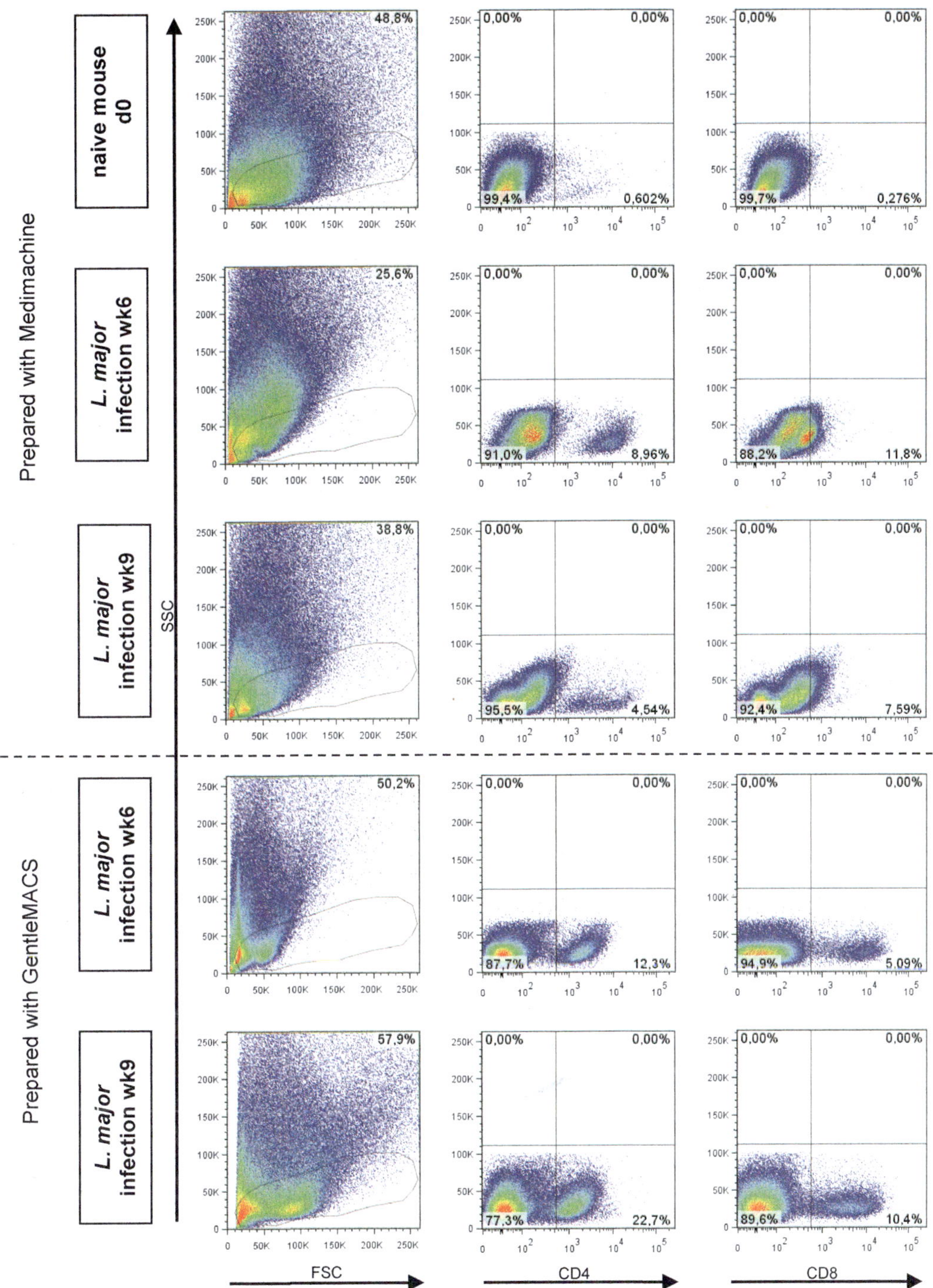


**Fig. 3** Frequencies of skin-infiltrating T cells in *L. major* infections. Mice were infected with $2 \times 10^5$ *L. major* parasites. In week 6, inflammatory cells were harvested from infected ears using different devices. Representative FACS stainings are depicted

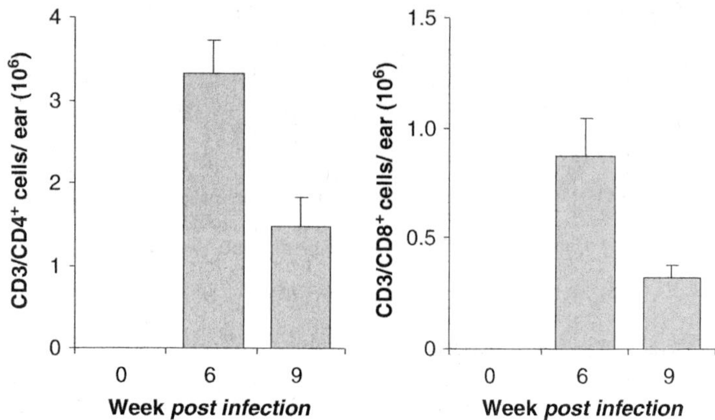


**Fig. 4** T cell numbers isolated from infected skin over time. Ears of *L. major-infected* mice were harvested at the indicated time points and T cell numbers calculated from total cell numbers and CD4/CD8 frequencies determined by FACS analysis (mean ± SEM, *n* = 3)

3. T cells can be restimulated with antigen using, e.g., CFSE labelling to determine antigen-specific T cell frequency (Fig. 5). Note that the frequency of isolated antigen-specific CD4 and CD8 T cells differed depending on the mechanical isolation device. In addition, in contrast to restimulated LN cells, in skin, IFNγ production of T cells as well as non-T cells was detected (prior studies suggested a role for NK cells in early IFNγ release in leishmaniasis).

## 4 Notes

1. Generally, in skin inflammatory processes, more acute infiltration with neutrophils and inflammatory monocytes as well as DC can be observed at earlier time points (hours to days post-initiation of inflammation), whereas stronger T cell infiltrates are seen at later time points (e.g., in contact allergy, 24–48 h later, in chronic inflammation after weeks).
2. In our hands, the Gentle MACS Dissociator provided more efficient results of T cell isolation compared to the Medimachine; both methods can however easily be established. With the Gentle MACS Dissociator, the overall cell yield was higher and the speed to the isolation process was quicker.
3. For maintaining good cell viability (e.g., neutrophils) and preventing monocytes and macrophages to adhere to plastic, work on ice.

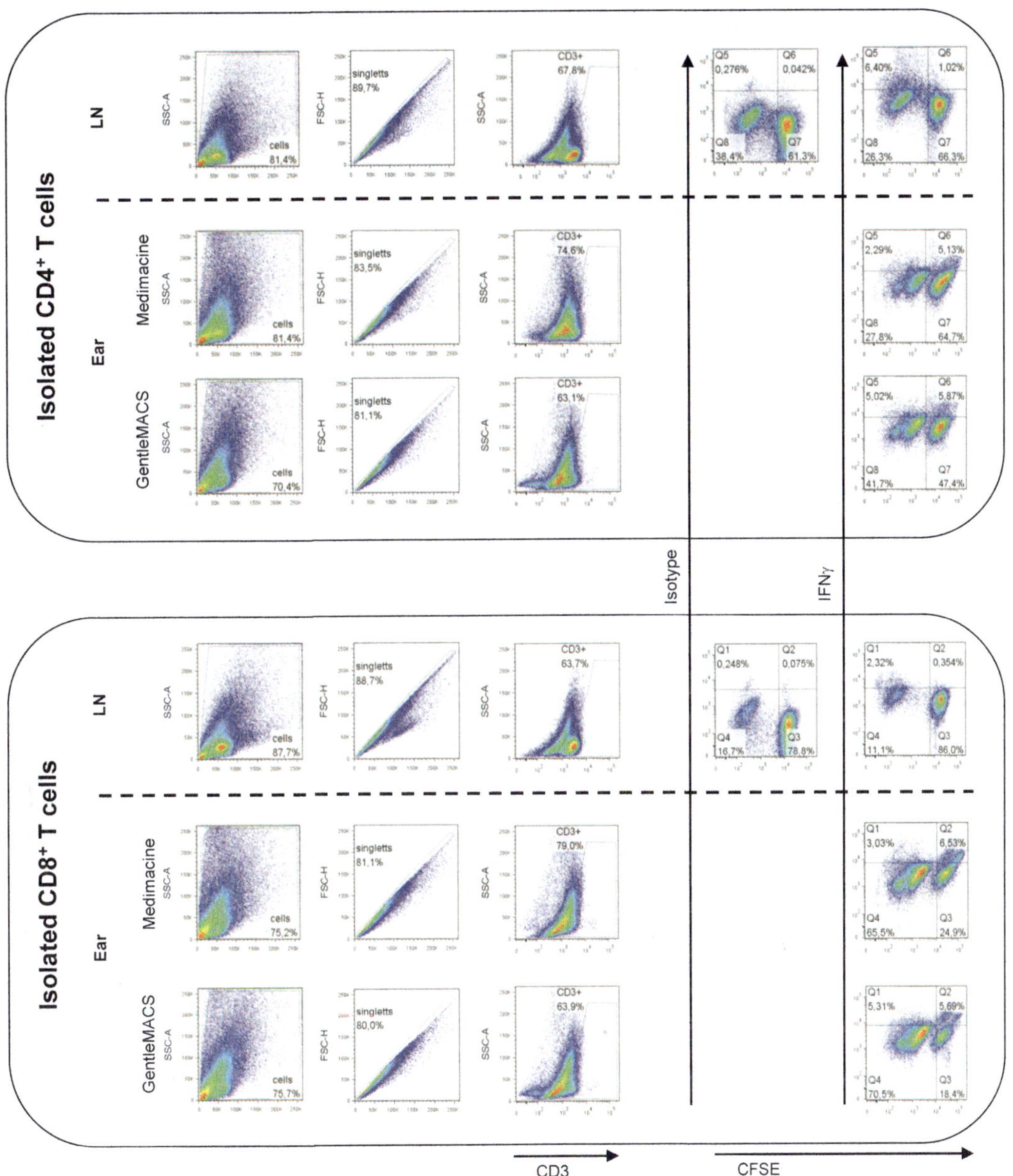


**Fig. 5** Proliferation and IFNγ release from isolated skin-inflammatory T cells. Mice were infected with *L. major*, ears and lymph nodes (LN) were harvested in week 6 post-infection. Inflammatory cells were isolated using the Gentle MACS. Subsequently, $CD8^+$ and $CD4^+$ T cells were isolated using microbeads. T cells were labelled with 1 μM CFSE and plated at $1 \times 10^6$ cells/200 μL in the presence of *Leishmania* antigen. On day 4, cells were harvested and stimulated with PMA/ionomycin using standard protocols. Representative stainings of ear and LN cells are shown

4. For detailed analyses, a pregating of T cells in FSC/SSC as shown in Fig. 2 may be required.
5. The protocol may be used for human tissue as well; specific modifications may be required.

**Table 1**

**Cell numbers harvested from ear skin after *L. major* infection**

| | Medimachine | | Gentle MACS | |
|---|---|---|---|---|
| Total cells | $76 \times 10^6$ | (4 ears) | $87 \times 10^6$ | (5 ears) |
| 1. Step: Anti-CD8 beads | $8 \times 10^5$ | 1.1 % | $10 \times 10^5$ | 1.1 % |
| 2. Step: Anti-CD4 beads | $8 \times 10^5$ | 1.1 % | $15 \times 10^5$ | 1.7 % |

C57BL/6 mice were infected with $2 \times 10^5$ *L. major* parasites. Ears were harvested in week 6 and cells isolated using the protocols described. $CD8^+$ and $CD4^+$ T cells were subsequently enriched from the suspensions using microbeads and the manufacturer's instructions

## 5 Summary

Isolation of T cells from murine (and human) skin can be accomplished with ease and high reproducibly using a robust experimental setup based on enzymatic predigestion of skin followed by mechanical disruption. Using this protocol, reasonably high cell numbers can be isolated followed by additional steps for an in-depth characterization of skin-infiltrating T cells.

## Acknowledgements

The present work was supported by GK1043, DFG STE 833/6-2, STE 833/11-1, and STE 833/12-1.

### References

1. Clark RA, Chong B, Mirchandani N, Brinster NK, Yamanaka K, Dowgiert RK, Kupper TS (2006) The vast majority of CLA+ T cells are resident in normal skin. J Immunol 176(7): 4431–4439
2. Kupper TS, Fuhlbrigge RC (2004) Immune surveillance in the skin: mechanisms and clinical consequences. Nat Rev Immunol 4: 211–222
3. Berg D, Otley CC (2002) Skin cancer in organ transplant recipients: epidemiology, pathogenesis, and management. J Am Acad Dermatol 47:1–17
4. Boyman O, Hefti HP, Conrad C, Nickoloff BJ, Suter M, Nestle FO (2004) Spontaneous development of psoriasis in a new animal model shows an essential role for resident T cells and tumor necrosis factor-α. J Exp Med 199:731–736
5. Steward-Tharp SM, Song YJ, Siegel RM, O'Shea JJ (2010) New insights into T cell biology and T cell-directed therapy for autoimmunity, inflammation, and immunosuppression. Ann N Y Acad Sci 1183:123–148
6. Clark RA (2010) Skin-resident T, cells: the ups and downs of on site immunity. J Invest Dermatol 130(2):362–370
7. Ghoreschi K, Laurence A, Yang XP, Hirahara K, O'Shea JJ (2011) T helper 17 cell heterogeneity and pathogenicity in autoimmune disease. Trends Immunol 32(9):395–401
8. Waisman A (2012) To be 17 again–anti-interleukin-17 treatment for psoriasis. N Engl J Med 366(13):1251–1252
9. Martin SF (2012) Allergic contact dermatitis: xenoinflammation of the skin. Curr Opin Immunol 24(6):720–729

10. Eming SA, Hammerschmidt M, Krieg T, Roers A (2009) Interrelation of immunity and tissue repair or regeneration. Semin Cell Dev Biol 20(5):517–527
11. Maurer M, Dondji B, von Stebut E (2009) What determines the success or failure of intracellular cutaneous parasites? Lessons learned from leishmaniasis. Med Microbiol Immunol 198(3):137–146
12. Dudda JC, Simon JC, Martin S (2004) Dendritic cell immunization route determines CD8+ T cell trafficking to inflamed skin: role for tissue microenvironment and dendritic cells in establishment of T cell-homing subsets. J Immunol 172(2):857–863
13. Belkaid Y, Hoffmann KF, Mendez S, Kamhawi S, Udey MC, Wynn TA, Sacks DL (2001) The role of interleukin (IL)-10 in the persistence of Leishmania major in the skin after healing and the therapeutic potential of anti-IL-10 receptor antibody for sterile cure. J Exp Med 194(10):1497–1506
14. Woelbing F et al (2006) Uptake of Leishmania major by dendritic cells is mediated by Fcγ receptors and facilitates acquisition of protective immunity. J Exp Med 203:177–188
15. Kautz-Neu K et al (2011) Langerhans cells are important negative regulators of the anti-Leishmania response. J Exp Med 208:885–891
16. Ludwig RJ, Bergmann P, Garbaraviciene J, von Stebut E, Radeke HH, Gille J, Diehl S, Hardt K, Henschler R, Kaufmann R, Pfeilschifter JM, Boehncke WH (2010) Platelet, not endothelial, P-selectin expression contributes to generation of immunity in cutaneous contact hypersensitivity. Am J Pathol 176(3):1339–1345

# Chapter 2

# Isolation of Leukocytes from Mouse Central Nervous System


## Iva Lelios and Melanie Greter



## Abstract

During neuroinflammatory or neurodegenerative diseases, it is often critical to characterize the composition of infiltrating immune cells. This protocol describes a reliable, fast, and simple method for the isolation of leukocytes from murine central nervous system (CNS) during steady state or inflammation for analysis by flow cytometry or other techniques.



**Key words** Central nervous system (CNS), Immune cell isolation from CNS, Percoll gradient, Flow cytometry, Collagenase treatment, Microglia, Neuroinflammation, Brain, Lymphocytes, Myeloid cells


## 1 Introduction

Under many pathological CNS conditions, immune cells such as lymphocytes, neutrophils, monocytes, and macrophages invade the brain and spinal cord. While histological analysis is ideal to localize a CNS lesion and to provide insight into the qualitative pathology of a CNS disease, precise and quantitative characterization of the immune composite is not easily achievable. This mainly stems from the fact that several cell surface markers are needed for the identification of the different immune cells, especially for the various myeloid cell populations during an inflammation [1]. Here we describe an efficient protocol to remove myelin debris in order to obtain a single-cell suspension enriched for $CD45^+$ cells using a Percoll gradient [2, 3]. These cells can then be processed for further procedures, for example in vitro cultures, analysis of cytokine profiles, RT-PCR analysis for mRNA expression, or staining with antibodies for flow cytometry. Flow cytometry allows the complex simultaneous analysis of many different cell surface and activation markers, transcription factors, and intracellular cytokine stainings. The method described here is not only useful for the analysis of CNS-infiltrating immune cells but is also valuable for the isolation and examination of microglia under


Ari Waisman and Burkhard Becher (eds.), *T-Helper Cells: Methods and Protocols*, Methods in Molecular Biology, vol. 1193, DOI 10.1007/978-1-4939-1212-4_2, © Springer Science+Business Media New York 2014

physiological conditions. Microglia are the resident macrophages of the CNS and represent a small percentage of all cells in the brain [4]. With this protocol, 50–80 % of $CD45^+$ cells isolated from normal brains will be microglia.

## 2 Materials

- Collagenase type 4 from *Clostridium histolyticum* (Sigma).
- Phosphate-buffered saline (PBS), pH 7.4.
- Fetal calf serum (FCS).
- Hanks' balanced salt solution (HBSS) with $CaCl_2$ and $MgCl_2$ (Gibco).
- 6-Well tissue culture plates.
- 3-mL syringe.
- 18 G × 1½ needle.
- 50 mL Falcon tubes.
- Percoll (GE Healthcare Life Sciences).
- Cell strainer (70 μm).
- Fixed-angle rotor centrifuge.

## 3 Methods

1. Before starting prepare collagenase solution:
   Dissolve collagenase type IV from *Clostridium histolyticum* to a concentration of 0.4 mg/mL in HBSS containing 10 % FCS.
2. Anesthetize mice deeply.
3. Open chest cavity and perfuse mice transcardially with ice-cold PBS to remove all circulating leukocytes and red blood cells from the CNS.
4. Dissect brain and spinal cord (*see* **Note 1**).
5. Transfer brain and spinal cord into 4 mL collagenase solution in a 6-well plate.
6. Cut the tissue into small pieces using small dissection scissors (*see* **Note 2**).
7. Incubate at 37 °C for 45 min.
8. Homogenize the cell suspension by passing it several times through a 3-mL syringe with a 18 × 1½ G needle.
9. Filter the cell suspension through a 70 μm cell strainer into 50 mL Falcon tube.

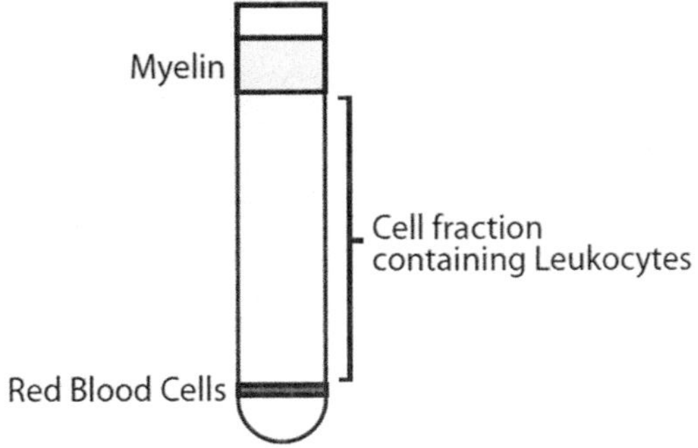


**Fig. 1** After centrifugation of the Percoll suspension, carefully collect the leukocyte-containing fraction

10. To wash the cell suspension, add 20 mL of PBS and centrifuge at 450 × *g*, 4 °C, for 5 min.
11. Discard the supernatant carefully.
12. Resuspend the pellet in PBS to a volume of 10.5 mL. Add 4.5 mL of Percoll and mix by pipetting up and down.
13. Centrifuge the suspension using a fixed-angle rotor at 15,000 × *g*, 4 °C, for 30 min.

    Important: Set centrifuge brake to 0.
14. After centrifugation, three layers will have formed (*see* Fig. 1).
15. Using a vacuum pump or a pipette, carefully remove the topmost layer, which contains myelin.
16. Filter the remaining suspension through a 70 μm cell strainer into a 50 mL Falcon tube (*see* **Notes 3** and **4**).
17. Fill the tube up with PBS and centrifuge at 450 × *g*, 4 °C, for 5 min.
18. Discard the supernatant. Resuspend the pellet in 1 mL PBS. Proceed with further processing (e.g., antibody staining for flow cytometry).
19. For flow cytometry analysis, *see* Chapters 5 and 6. Markers useful to analyze the different CNS leukocyte populations are described in Table 1. An example for a gating strategy for flow cytometry analysis is shown in Fig. 2 of a normal mouse and an EAE mouse (*see* **Note 5**).

## 4 Notes

1. Spinal cord isolation: After decapitation, make a perpendicular cut through the spinal column at the base of the spinal cord. Insert a 20 mL syringe (18 G × 1½ needle) filled with PBS into

**Table 1**

**Summarizes an example of markers to classify leukocytes in the steady-state or the inflamed CNS**

| Steady state | | | Inflammation | | | |
|---|---|---|---|---|---|---|
| **Microglia** | **Macrophages** | **Dendritic cells** | **B cells** | **T cells** | **Monocytes/moDCs** | **Neutrophils** |
| $CD45^{lo}$ | $CD45^{hi}$ | $CD45^{hi}$ | $CD45^{hi}$ | $CD45^{hi}$ | $CD45^{hi}$ | $CD45^{hi}$ |
| $CD11b^{+}$ | $CD11b^{+}$ | $MHCII^{+}$ | $B220^{+}$ | $CD3^{+}$ | $CD11b^{+}$ | $CD11b^{+}$ |
| $F4/80^{+}$ $CD64^{+}$ | $F4/80^{+}$ $CD64^{+}$ | $CD11c^{+}$ $CD11b^{+}$ or $CD103^{+}$ | $CD19^{+}$ | $CD4^{+}$ or $CD8^{+}$ | $F4/80^{+}$ $Ly6C^{-/+}$ $MHCII^{-/+}$ $CD11c^{-/+}$ | $Ly6G^{+}$ |

In the steady-state CNS, the majority of $CD45^{+}$ cells are microglia, which can be distinguished from perivascular macrophages by the levels of CD45 expression (microglia are $CD45^{lo}$ whereas other leukocytes are $CD45^{hi}$). In the inflamed CNS, an increase in immune cells ($CD45^{hi}$) can be detected
*MoDCs* monocyte-derived dendritic cells

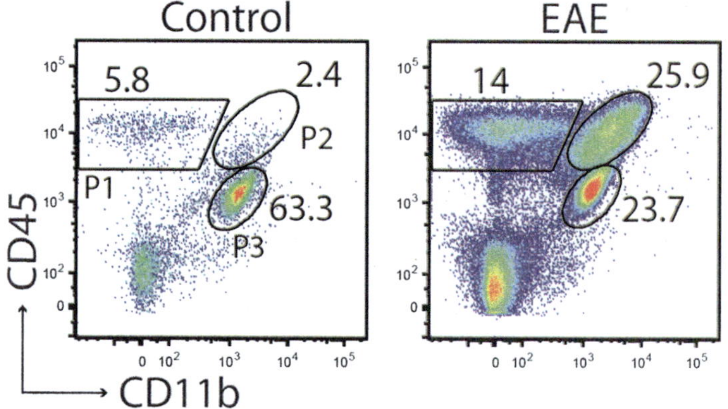


**Fig. 2** Flow cytometry analysis of CNS cells isolated from an EAE-diseased mouse and a healthy control mouse. Percentage of each population is indicated next to the gate. $CD45^{lo}CD11b^{+}$ cells represent microglia (P3). Note the infiltrating $CD45^{hi}$ cells in the EAE brain. $CD45^{hi}CD11b^{+}$ myeloid cells (P2) can be further subdivided into monocytes, neutrophils, inflammatory DCs, and macrophages (*see* Table 1 for specific markers). The majority of $CD45^{hi}CD11b^{-}$ cells are T and B cells (P1)

the spinal canal at the base. Apply pressure with your fingers on the column at the base and flush the spinal cord out.

2. For cutting, the tissue can be transferred to a 2 mL Eppendorf tube without any liquid. After cutting with pointed scissors inside the Eppendorf tube, the pieces are transferred back to the collagenase-containing well.
3. If the mice were not well perfused, a layer of red blood cells will form at the bottom of the tube after the centrifugation (Fig. 1). In this case, do not collect the bottom layer.

4. White myelin-containing cell clumps can sometimes be found in this fraction. These clumps are easily removed with a pipette or while filtering the cell suspension through the cell strainer.
5. Experimental autoimmune encephalomyelitis (EAE) is the animal model for multiple sclerosis, which is an autoimmune, inflammatory, and demyelinating disease of the CNS [5]. EAE can be induced in susceptible mouse strains by immunization with myelin proteins/peptides in complete Freund's adjuvant (CFA) or by the transfer of myelin-reactive $CD4^+$ T cells.

## References

1. Prinz M, Priller J, Sisodia SS, Ransohoff RM (2011) Heterogeneity of CNS myeloid cells and their roles in neurodegeneration. Nat Neurosci 14:1227
2. Dick AD, Ford AL, Forrester JV, Sedgwick JD (1995) Flow cytometric identification of a minority population of MHC class II positive cells in the normal rat retina distinct from CD45lowCD11b/c+CD4low parenchymal microglia. Br J Ophthalmol 79:834
3. Greter M et al (2005) Dendritic cells permit immune invasion of the CNS in an animal model of multiple sclerosis. Nat Med 11:328
4. Ransohoff RM, Cardona AE (2010) The myeloid cells of the central nervous system parenchyma. Nature 468:253
5. Schreiner B, Heppner FL, Becher B (2009) Modeling multiple sclerosis in laboratory animals. Semin Immunopathol 31:479

# Chapter 3

# Isolation of T Cells from the Gut

**Sonja Reißig, Christopher Hackenbruch, and Nadine Hövelmeyer**

## Abstract

The lymphocytes of epithelial and lamina proprial compartments of the intestine are phenotypically and functionally distinct and serve a wide range of functions in the intestinal mucosa like regulating intestinal homeostasis, maintaining epithelial barrier function as well as regulating adaptive and innate immune responses. To analyze the role of these cells in different disease states, it is necessary to isolate pure cell populations of the intraepithelial lymphocytes (IEL) and lamina propria lymphocytes (LPL) of the gut. In this protocol we describe a method to isolate T cells from IEL and LPL, which can be used for further investigations like comparative studies of mRNA expression, cell proliferation assay, or protein analysis.

**Key words** Mucosal immunology, Lamina propria, Gut, T cells, Lamina propria lymphocytes, Intraepithelial lymphocytes

## 1 Introduction

The intestinal mucosal immune system actively contributes to the maintenance of mucosal homeostasis and defends against pathogenic microbes. It consists of three major lymphoid areas: (1) the lamina propria (LP) which lies just beneath the basement membrane in the intestinal villi and contains the lamina propria lymphocytes (LPL); (2) the intraepithelial compartment which is located just above the basement membrane between the columnar epithelial cells and comprises the intraepithelial lymphocytes (IEL); (3) the Peyer's patches (PP) which are organized in lymphoid nodules (akin to lymph nodes) embedded in the gut wall, separated from the LP and IEL. The LP, PP, and IEL lymphoid populations form a complex, interconnected network that responds to immunological insults in the intestine. Therefore, these lymphocyte populations should be analyzed when studying the immunological status of the intestine.

Various techniques have been described so far for the isolation of intestinal cells [1, 2]. IEL fractions have been isolated by gentle mechanical manipulation [3], by EDTA treatment [4–6], and by enzymatic treatment [7].

Ari Waisman and Burkhard Becher (eds.), *T-Helper Cells: Methods and Protocols*, Methods in Molecular Biology, vol. 1193, DOI 10.1007/978-1-4939-1212-4_3, 

In the present protocol, we describe a simple modification of a standard lamina propria lymphocyte and intraepithelial lymphocyte isolation technique [8] that involves the combination of mechanical dissociation with enzymatic degradation of the extracellular adhesion proteins. The protocol can be used to characterize T cell subpopulations isolated from LPL and/or IEL of the colon or of the small intestines or subparts of it like the duodenum, jejunum, or ileum. The isolated cells should be used directly for downstream applications such as magnetic cell separation for T cells, cellular or molecular analysis.

The stated volumes in this protocol are calculated for one intestine, either small intestine or colon. Do not pool the small intestine and colon for the purification procedure.

## 2 Materials

### 2.1 Equipment

1. Scissors.
2. Forceps.
3. Petri dishes.
4. 100 μm cell strainer.
5. 5 and 50 mL Falcon conical centrifugation tubes.
6. gentleMACS™ tubes (alternatively use 50 mL Falcon conical centrifugation tubes).
7. gentleMACS dissociator (alternatively use vortexer).
8. Vortexer.
9. Centrifuge used in cell culture.
10. Thermal incubator with rotation unit.
11. PIPETBOY.

### 2.2 Reagent Setup

1. Predigestion solution: 1× HBSS (without $Ca^{2+}$ and $Mg^{2+}$, no Phenol Red) containing 10 mM HEPES, 5 mM EDTA, 1 mM DTT, and 5 % fetal calf serum (FCS).
2. Digestion solution: 1× HBSS (with $Ca^{2+}$ and $Mg^{2+}$, no Phenol Red) containing 10 mM HEPES, 0.5 mg/mL Collagenase D, 0.5 mg/mL DNase I grade II, 3 mg/mL Dispase II, and 5 % FCS. Prepare the digestion solution just before use.
3. 1× HBSS (without $Ca^{2+}$ and $Mg^{2+}$, no Phenol Red) with 5 % FCS.
4. Fluorescence-activated cell sorting (FACS) buffer: 2 % FCS in 1× PBS.
5. T cell medium: RPMI 1640 supplemented with 10 % FCS (decomplemented), 1 mM sodium pyruvate, 2 mM L-glutamine, 1× nonessential amino acids, 0.1 mM 2-β-mercaptoethanol, and 10 mM HEPES.

6. Percoll gradient 40 %: Use 42.01 mL of Percoll separation solution with 1.124 g/L density and dilute with 57.99 mL of 1× PBS.
7. Percoll gradient 80 %: Use 79.83 mL of Percoll separation solution with 1.124 g/L density and dilute with 20.17 mL of 1× PBS.
8. Sterile 1× PBS (without $Ca^{2+}$ and $Mg^{2+}$).

## 3 Methods

1. Sacrifice mice, remove the intestine, and place it in ice-cold 1× PBS in a petri dish (*see* **Note 1**).
2. Clear the intestine of feces by holding it with forceps and flushing with a 1 mL syringe filled with ice-cold 1× PBS.
3. Remove residual mesenteric fat tissue, excise Peyer's patches carefully (*see* **Note 2**), and open the intestine longitudinally.
4. Cut the intestine into 0.5–1 cm pieces, transfer them into a 50 mL tube, and wash them several times by vortexing in ice-cold 1× PBS until the buffer appears clean.
5. Transfer the tissue pieces into a new 50 mL tube containing 20 mL of pre-digestion solution (*see* **Notes 3** and **4**) and incubate sample for 20 min at 37 °C with slow rotation (40 × *g*) on a horizontal tube rotator.
6. After the incubation remove the epithelial cell layer, containing the IEL, by intensive vortexing for 10 s and passing through a 100 μm cell strainer placed on a 50 mL Falcon tube. The flow-through contains the IEL and can be stored on ice for the isolation of IEL.
7. Transfer the tissue pieces into a new 50 mL Falcon tube containing new 20 mL of the pre-digestion solution and incubate a second time for 20 min at 37 °C with slow rotation (40 × *g*) on a horizontal tube rotator.
8. After the incubation mix the samples by intensive vortexing for 10 s and pass the sample through a 100 μm cell strainer placed on a 50 mL Falcon tube.
9. Transfer the tissue pieces into a new 50 mL Falcon tube containing 10 mL HBSS with 5 % FCS for 10 min at 37 °C with rotation on a horizontal tube rotator.
10. After the incubation mix the samples by intensive vortexing for 10 s and pass the sample through a 100 μm cell strainer placed on a 50 mL Falcon tube.

    If IEL isolation is desired, pool the supernatants of all pre-digestion treatments and the washing step. Wash once with FACS buffer and store them on ice (*see* **Notes 5** and **6**).

11. Transfer the intestine tissue pieces into a petri dish and cut them in 1 mm$^2$ pieces using scissors or razor blades. Place the remaining tissue in gentleMACS™ tubes and add 2.5 mL digestion solution. Incubate the samples at 37 °C for 30 min with rotation on a horizontal tube rotator (*see* **Note 7**).
12. Dissociate the LPL with the gentleMACS dissociator by running the program lamina propria. After termination of the program, add 10 mL of FACS buffer to each sample and isolate the cells by passing through a 100 μm cell strainer.
13. Wash the cell strainer with 10 mL of FACS buffer. Centrifuge the cell suspension for 10 min at 300 × *g*, discard the supernatant, and resuspend cells in FACS buffer and store them on ice.
14. Use cells immediately for further experiments, for example for T cell magnetic cell separation or flow cytometry.
15. For purification of lymphocytes resuspend LPL or IEL in 4 mL of the 40 % fraction of a 40:80 Percoll gradient, and overlay them carefully on 8 mL of the 80 % fraction in a 15 mL Falcon tube.
16. Perform Percoll gradient separation by centrifugation for 20 min at 1,000 × *g* at room temperature without brakes.
17. After the centrifugation, LPL or IEL should be visible in a white ring at the interphase of the two different Percoll solutions. Collect the cells carefully and transfer them into a new 15 mL Falcon tube. Add FACS buffer and centrifuge the samples for 10 min at 300 × *g* at 20 °C.
18. Resuspend the cells directly in FACS buffer or T cell medium and store them on ice.

    Use the cells immediately for experiments, for example for flow cytometry or T cell magnetic cell separation. The isolated T cells can be used for comparative stimulation assays, proliferation assays, RNA extraction, or protein isolation.

## 4 Notes

1. Small intestines are considered from the beginning of the duodenum/pylorus to the caecum. Colon is considered from the caecum to the anus. To extract the whole colon break the pelvis laterally.
2. Peyer's patches are found only in the small intestines. Remove Peyer's patches before cleaning the intestine, because otherwise it might be hard to identify the Peyer's patches.
3. Preheat the pre-digestion solution to 37 °C before adding to the tissue.
4. Per digestion a volume of 40 mL of the pre-digestion is required.

5. In the meantime: Preheat the digestion solution to 37 °C before adding to the tissue.
6. Per digestion a volume of 2.5 mL of the digestion solution is required.
7. Alternatively: If you do not use the gentleMACS dissociator, place in **step 11** the tissue in a 50 mL Falcon tube for the digestion step. After the incubation time (**step 12**), vortex the Falcon tube intensively for 20 s and pass the cell solution through a 100 μm cell strainer set over a 50 mL Falcon tube. Ideally, all tissue pieces should be digested to invisible pieces.

## References


1. Bull DM, Bookman MA (1977) Isolation and functional characterization of human intestinal mucosal lymphoid cells. J Clin Invest 59: 966–974
2. Fiocchi C, Battisto JR, Farmer RG (1979) Gut mucosal lymphocytes in inflammatory bowel disease: isolation and preliminary functional characterization. Dig Dis Sci 24:705–717
3. Lundqvist C, Hammarstrom ML, Athlin L, Hammarstrom S (1992) Isolation of functionally active intraepithelial lymphocytes and enterocytes from human small and large intestine. J Immunol Methods 152: 253–263
4. Davies MD, Parrott DM (1981) Preparation and purification of lymphocytes from the epithelium and lamina propria of murine small intestine. Gut 22:481–488
5. Dillon SB, MacDonald TT (1984) Functional properties of lymphocytes isolated from murine small intestinal epithelium. Immunology 52:501–509
6. Mosley RL, Klein JR (1992) A rapid method for isolating murine intestine intraepithelial lymphocytes with high yield and purity. J Immunol Methods 156:19–26
7. Lefrancois L, Lycke N (2001) Isolation of mouse small intestinal intraepithelial lymphocytes, Peyer's patch, and lamina propria cells. In: Coligan JE et al (eds) Current protocols in immunology. Wiley, New York, NY, Chapter 3: Unit 3 19
8. Weigmann B, Tubbe I, Seidel D, Nicolaev A, Becker C et al (2007) Isolation and subsequent analysis of murine lamina propria mononuclear cells from colonic tissue. Nat Protoc 2:2307–2311

# Chapter 4

# T Cell Isolation from Mouse Kidneys


## Isis Ludwig-Portugall and Christian Kurts



## Abstract

The kidneys contain very few lymphocytes under homeostatic conditions. One kidney from a healthy mouse per average contains only $1–5 \times 10^3$ $CD4^+$ T cells. In immune-mediated kidney disease, γδ T cells, NKT cells, $CD4^+$ T cells, $CD8^+$ T cells, and regulatory T cells (Treg) infiltrate the kidney. Their numbers and subset composition of infiltrating T cells varies between the different forms of nephritis. For example, in glomerulonephritis $CD4^+$ T cells mediate renal injury, by local cytokine production, effector cell activation and/or by helping B cells to produce nephritogenic antibodies. A better understanding of the pathomechanisms of immune-mediated kidney diseases requires a method to isolate T cells from the kidney for ex vivo analysis. Here we describe an effective and specific isolation protocol for T cells from the murine kidney.



**Key words** Perfusion, DNAse and collagenase digestion, Magnetic cell separation, T cell sorting


## 1 Introduction

T cells play an important role in glomerulonephritis (GN), a group of several immune-mediated kidney diseases that initially target the renal glomeruli. T cells act either as helper cells for the production of nephritogenic T cells in lymphatic tissues or as effector cells within the kidney by cytokine production, by stimulation of macrophages or by intrinsic effector functions [1]. Tubulointerstitial T cell infiltrates are seen in many forms of GN [2–4]. The degree of infiltration correlates with disease progression in the most common form of GN, IgA nephropathy [5]. Immunosuppressive treatment is the therapy of choice in many forms of GN, although it is not always effective. Successful therapies often involve drugs that suppress T cell responses, like cyclosporine A. Harmful T cells are often differentiated as Th1 cells, or, as shown by recent studies, also by Th17 cells [6, 7]. In addition to these injurious T cells, regulatory T cells [8–10] can modify GN progression, although it is unknown whether these act within the kidney or in lymphatic tissues where nephritogenic Th1 and Th17 cells are primed. Moreover, also innate lymphocytes have been implicated in GN,


Ari Waisman and Burkhard Becher (eds.), *T-Helper Cells: Methods and Protocols*, Methods in Molecular Biology, vol. 1193, DOI 10.1007/978-1-4939-1212-4_4, © Springer Science+Business Media New York 2014

such as γδ T cells [11] or NKT cells [12]. Finally, T cells contribute not only to GN but also to interstitial nephritis.

Despite much efforts, the immune-mechanisms of GN remain incompletely understood. The elucidation of the role of T cells depends on the ability to isolate functional lymphocytes from the kidney. Here we describe a simple, efficient, and effective method to isolate these cells in a functional state from murine kidneys.

## 2 Materials

Always prepare the digestion medium on the day of the experiment and whilst working store all reagents on ice (unless otherwise indicated).

### 2.1 Perfusion

The following materials are required to perform a perfusion on murine kidneys:

1. Perfusion pump: for example the Masterflex L/S pump (Cole Parmer Instrument Company) as depicted in Fig. 1.
2. Kidneys can be perfused at a perfusion rate between 3.2 and 4.0 mL/min and the tubing size on the machine is 14, which is the actual diameter of the tube.
3. The machine is first primed using freshly prepared perfusion solution (sterile PBS) at room temperature.
4. The perfusion machine is connected to the mouse using a 0.45 × 12 mm gauge needle which is attached to the tube (*see* Fig. 1).

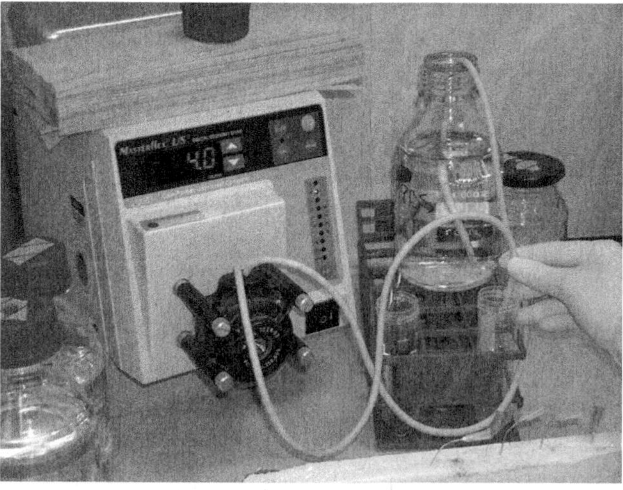


**Fig. 1** Perfusion pump composition with perfusion solution and tube with the attached injection needle

### 2.2 Solutions

#### 2.2.1 Digestion Buffer

RPMI 1640 medium: 10 mg/mL Type 1 Collagenase, 10 mg/mL DNAse, 10 % FCS, 25 mM HEPES, 100 Units Penicillin, and 0.1 mg/mL Streptomycin.

#### 2.2.2 Digestion Stopping Buffer

RPMI 1640 medium: 2 % FCS.

#### 2.2.3 MACS Buffer

MACS buffer can be purchased from the firm or made according to the following recipe: PBS sterile: 0.5 % BSA and 2 mM EDTA.

### 2.3 Magnetic Cell Separation

There are various methods of magnetic cell sorting but here we shall focus on the system provided by Miltenyi Biotec (Bergisch Gladbach, Germany).

The firm offers kits to isolate the entire T cell population of the different subsets. This method gives a purification rate around 60–80 % but it is recommended to check the purity of the isolated cells with flow cytometry to ensure that you have purified the desired population.

### 2.4 T Cell Sorting

1. Before staining the T cells with Ab against their characteristic surface molecules, use CD45 MACS beads (Miltenyi, Germany) according to the manufacturers' instructions.
2. Keep cells in RPMI 1640 media for the staining with the Abs. The sorting of cells is necessary when a very pure population of cells is required.

## 3 Methods

The three different methods described here such as digestion, magnetic cell purification and cell sorting to purify T cells from the kidney should be chosen depending on the desired analysis. The digestion alone is good enough for analysis by flow cytometry, the magnetic cell purification is helpful for cell culture or adoptive transfer studies and the cell sorting is needed if DNA or RNA Arrays are performed.

### 3.1 Perfusion of the Kidney

Sometimes it is helpful to perfuse the kidney prior to lymphocyte preparation to remove leucocytes from the glomeruli. In addition, this allows one to analyze organ infiltrated lymphocytes as blood derived cells are washed out.

1. Prior to opening the abdominal area euthanized mice should be sprayed with ethanol.
2. After opening the abdominal cavity with sterile scissors and tweezers, the chest area is carefully opened but should remain intact without harming any blood vessels.

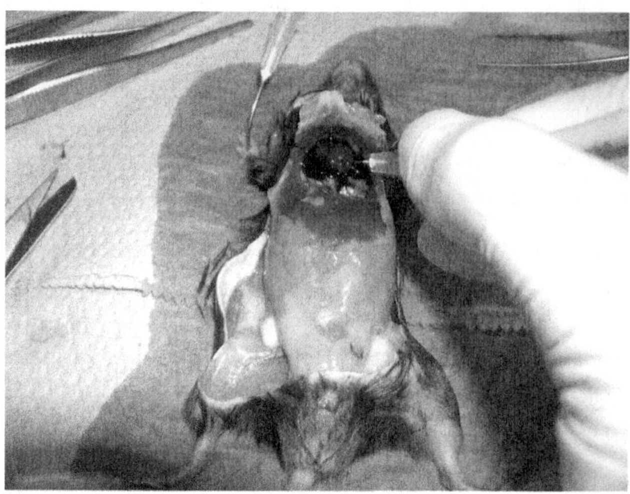

**Fig. 2** Application of the needle to perfuse the mouse

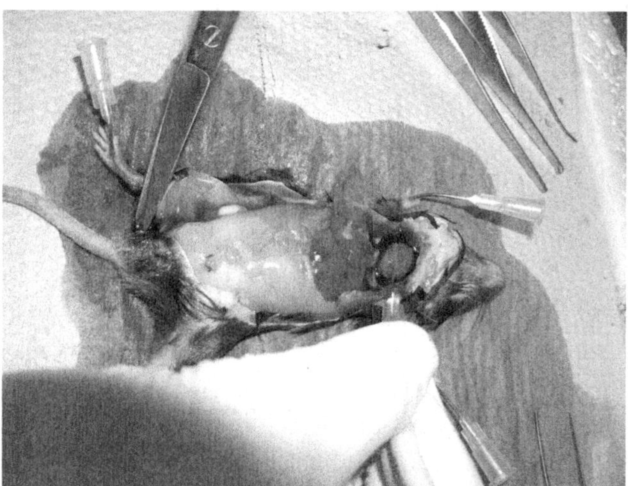

**Fig. 3** Perfused mouse. The efficiency is detectable by the color changes of the different organs

3. A small incision should then be made in the portal vein and a gauge needle attached to the pump should be carefully inserted into the left heart ventricle (Fig. 2).
4. This is followed by starting the pump which will flush the perfusion solution (PBS) through the cardiovascular system. An indication that the perfusion is working correctly can be seen via the color change to the liver (dark red to off-white).
5. At that time point a small incision on the leg artery is made using a scissor. This provides an exit for the waste fluids (as depicted in Fig. 3). Further help will be provided in the section "Notes".

### 3.2 Kidney Digestion and Preparation of Single Cell Suspension

The removal of the kidney capsule ensures proper digestion. The above described kidney perfusion (Subheading 3.1) enhances the isolation of infiltrating lymphocytes since it removes leucocytes from the glomeruli.

1. After removing the kidneys, detach the capsules and place the kidneys in a 24 well culture plate in 2 mL PBS on ice.
2. Next the kidneys are transferred into a fresh 24-well plate containing 2 mL of digestion media. Then, whilst holding the organ with sterile forceps 1 mL of the digestion media is injected into the kidney. Thereafter the kidney is mechanically disrupted into small pieces and the tissue is incubated at 37 °C for 30 min with gentle shaking on an orbital shaker.
3. After 30 min the kidney is further disrupted using a plunger from a 2 mL syringe and this procedure is followed by the incubation of the tissue for a further 20 min at 37 °C.
4. To stop digestion, 1 mL of RPMI 1640 media containing 2% FCS is added to the wells. Using a sterile 1 mL pipette the digestion mixture is homogenized until no tissue particles are visible.
5. In the next step the digested kidney is then transferred to a 15 mL Falcon tube, filtered through 100 mm nylon mesh to remove any remaining tissue fragments.
6. In a last step the wells of the plate are rinsed again with RPMI 1640 media and transferred into the 15 mL tube. Cell suspensions should be kept on ice until the next steps are performed. If cells are used for FACS analysis directly further help will be provided in the section "Notes".

### 3.3 Magnetic Bead Separation

This isolation can be performed by both negative selection (cells, not of interest, are labeled and retained in the column) or positive selection where the cells of interest are labeled and retained in the column attached to antibody conjugated magnetic beads.

For the isolation of Treg we recommend the Treg isolation kit from Miltenyi, which combines first a negative selection of CD4 T cells and then a positive selection of CD25+ cells.

For NKT cells a two step positive selection could be used which combines first CD1d-αGalCer Tetramer-PE staining with the detection of PE with anti-PE beads. Also γδ T cells could be magnetically separated by using a two-step positive selection kit from Miltenyi, but we recommend the cell sorting purification for NKT cells and γδ T cells to get a better purity of these cells. For the isolation of the kidney T cells ($CD4^+$ or $CD8^+$ T cells) we recommend the positive isolation method, which will deliver a purity of 60–80 % and is described in the following protocol.

1. Continuing from the digestion step (Subheading 3.2) the organ suspension is centrifuge at $250 \times g$ for 5 min and the

pellet is washed in MACS buffer. The cells are re-centrifuged and each kidney is resuspended in 300 μL MACS buffer.

2. The following protocol describes the procedure for a single kidney and positive selection by using 30 μL of T cell beads (Miltenyi Biotec) are added to each organ suspension and which is then carefully vortexed. The cell suspension is then incubated at 4 °C for 15 min.
3. Cell suspensions are then topped up with 5 mL MACS buffer, centrifuged at 200 × *g*, and the pellet is resuspended in 1 mL MACS buffer. During this time a large separation (LS) column is placed on the magnet and equilibrated with 3 mL MACS buffer as per the manufacturers' instructions.
4. Prior to separation it is recommended to pass the cell/bead suspension through a 50 mm nylon mesh filter, which can be placed on top of the column.
5. After the cell suspension has passed through the column by gravity the column should be washed three times with 2 mL MACS buffer.
6. In the end the positive selected T cells need to be detached from the column. Therefore the column is removed from the magnetic field and 2 mL MACS buffer is added to the column to wash the cells into a fresh 15 mL tube.
7. After the buffer has passed through the column the solution is then further centrifuged at 200 × *g* for 5 min to pellet the cells.
8. Afterwards the cells are and checked for purity by FACS (Fig. 4) and than resuspended for example in culture media for further applications.

### 3.4 T Cell Sorting by Flow Cytometry

It is advisable to pre-isolate renal T cells using the above described magnetic bead separation method using CD45 beads before sorting or especially CD1d-αGalCer Tetramer-PE staining + anti PE beads for NKT cells. Special recommendations for cells purification will be provided in the section "Notes". This removes other kidney cell fragments and prevents the sorter from clogging. Furthermore, it decreases the time required for the sort.

1. Following digestion, cells should be centrifuged at 200 × *g* for 5 min at 4 °C. The cell suspension should be then incubated with antibodies specific for the desired T cell populations and a typical cocktail could consist of CD45, CD3, CD4, or CD8 for conventional T cells or anti-TCR specific antibodies such as anti TCR-β and CD1d-αGalCer Tetramer (for NKT cells) or CD45, CD3, anti-γδ TCR (for γδ T cells) and Hoechst 33258.
2. After MACS purification the $CD45^+$ cells are further stained with the required T cell surface marker and afterwards

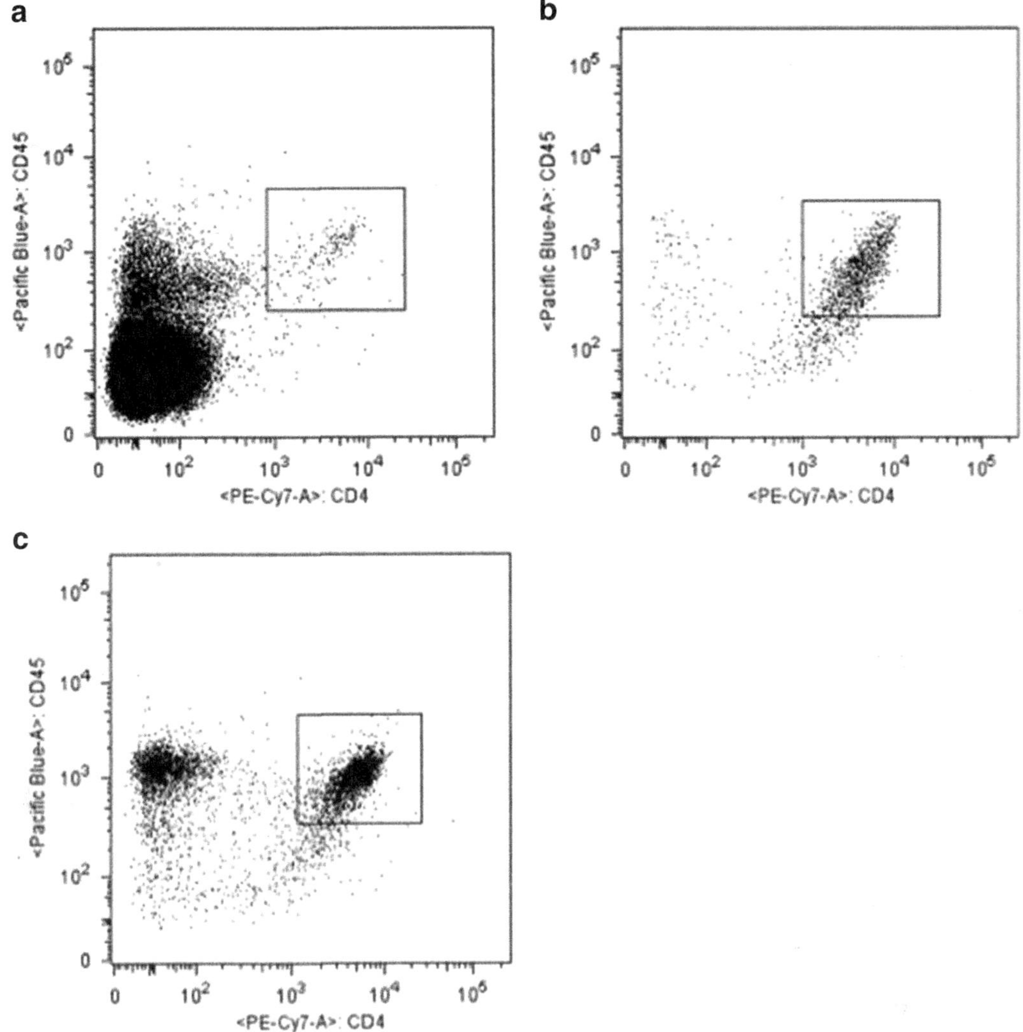


**Fig. 4** FACS dot blots after different purification steps. (**a**) After digestion, (**b**) after CD4 positive magnetic cell purification, and (**c**) after CD45 MACS before cell sorting

resuspended at a concentration of $5 \times 10^6$ cells/mL in culture medium. These cells are then sorted according to their fluorescent signal.

3. A cell population with a purity of 95–99 % can be typically obtained with cell sorting. After sorting, cells are washed in RPMI 1640 medium and can be used for further assays, e.g., DNA or RNA arrays, where a very pure population of cells is required or where very low numbers of the desired cells are contained in the kidney which reduces the efficiency of MACS separation.

## 4 Notes

1. Sometimes it is necessary during perfusion to cut the leg artery on the other leg as well.
2. It can take up to 10 min to get a good perfusion of the kidney which can also be monitored by the color change from dark red to pale pink.
3. For direct FACS analysis after kidney digestion it is beneficial to take up the kidney cell suspension in 4 mL Medium and let it rest for 4 min on ice. During this 4-min period the bigger tubular cells will settle to the bottom of the falcon and the immune cells will stay in solution and thereby can be transferred to a new falcon. Continue with the staining of the T cells with the Ab cocktail of choice.
4. The kidneys from individual mice can be pooled together for magnetic cell separation but then the volume of MACS buffer and magnetic cell separation beads will need adapting. Use only up to two kidneys on one LS column.
5. For a better purity during the positive separation of T cells, include two more washing steps of the column while the column is placed in the magnet, use MACS buffer with 4 mM EDTA and repeat the magnetic cell purification if necessary.
6. CD45 MACS purification prior to kidney cell sorting can help to reduce the sorting time, cells are more viable and Medium containing 4 mM EDTA can help to avoid plugging of the sorter.
7. Purification of NKT cells or γδ T cells from the kidney should be done by a combination of magnetic cell preparation and cell sorting to achieve a higher purity.

## Acknowledgements

We would like to acknowledge the DFG who is founding a project for I.L.-P. and C.K. (LU 1387/2-1).

### References

1. Kurts C, Heymann F, Lukacs-Kornek V, Boor P, Floege J (2007) Role of T cells and dendritic cells in glomerular immunopathology. Semin Immunopathol 29:317–335
2. Couzi L, Merville P, Deminiere C, Moreau JF, Combe C, Pellegrin JL, Viallard JF, Blanco P (2007) Predominance of CD8+ T lymphocytes among periglomerular infiltrating cells and link to the prognosis of class III and class IV lupus nephritis. Arthritis Rheum 56:2362–2370
3. Foster MH (2007) T cells and B cells in lupus nephritis. Semin Nephrol 27:47–58
4. Masutani K, Akahoshi M, Tsuruya K, Tokumoto M, Ninomiya T, Kohsaka T, Fukuda

K, Kanai H, Nakashima H, Otsuka T, Hirakata H (2001) Predominance of Th1 immune response in diffuse proliferative lupus nephritis. Arthritis Rheum 44:2097–2106

5. Falk MC, Ng G, Zhang GY, Fanning GC, Roy LP, Bannister KM, Thomas AC, Clarkson AR, Woodroffe AJ, Knight JF (1995) Infiltration of the kidney by alpha beta and gamma delta T cells: effect on progression in IgA nephropathy. Kidney Int 47:177–185
6. Ooi JD, Kitching AR, Holdsworth SR (2010) Review: T helper 17 cells: their role in glomerulonephritis. Nephrology (Carlton) 15:513–521
7. Paust HJ, Turner JE, Riedel JH, Disteldorf E, Peters A, Schmidt T, Krebs C, Velden J, Mittrucker HW, Steinmetz OM, Stahl RA, Panzer U (2012) Chemokines play a critical role in the cross-regulation of Th1 and Th17 immune responses in murine crescentic glomerulonephritis. Kidney Int 82:72–83
8. Ooi JD, Snelgrove SL, Engel DR, Hochheiser K, Ludwig-Portugall I, Nozaki Y, O'Sullivan KM, Hickey MJ, Holdsworth SR, Kurts C, Kitching AR (2011) Endogenous foxp3(+) T-regulatory cells suppress anti-glomerular basement membrane nephritis. Kidney Int 79:977–986
9. Paust HJ, Ostmann A, Erhardt A, Turner JE, Velden J, Mittrucker HW, Sparwasser T, Panzer U, Tiegs G (2011) Regulatory T cells control the Th1 immune response in murine crescentic glomerulonephritis. Kidney Int 80:154–164
10. Wolf D, Hochegger K, Wolf AM, Rumpold HF, Gastl G, Tilg H, Mayer G, Gunsilius E, Rosenkranz AR (2005) CD4+CD25+ regulatory T cells inhibit experimental anti-glomerular basement membrane glomerulonephritis in mice. J Am Soc Nephrol 16:1360–1370
11. Turner JE, Krebs C, Tittel AP, Paust HJ, Meyer-Schwesinger C, Bennstein SB, Steinmetz OM, Prinz I, Magnus T, Korn T, Stahl RA, Kurts C, Panzer U (2012) IL-17A production by renal gammadelta T cells promotes kidney injury in crescentic GN. J Am Soc Nephrol 23:1486–1495
12. Riedel JH, Paust HJ, Turner JE, Tittel AP, Krebs C, Disteldorf E, Wegscheid C, Tiegs G, Velden J, Mittrucker HW, Garbi N, Stahl RA, Steinmetz OM, Kurts C, Panzer U (2012) Immature renal dendritic cells recruit regulatory CXCR6(+) invariant natural killer T cells to attenuate crescentic GN. J Am Soc Nephrol 23:1987–2000

# Part II

## Analysis of T Cell Function and Phenotypes

# Chapter 5

# Intracellular Staining for Cytokines and Transcription Factors


## Florian Mair and Vinko Tosevski



## Abstract

Within the past years immune cells in general and T cells in particular have been categorized into a vast variety of subsets with different functional properties. One of the key technologies fueling this emerging complexity is intracellular staining for effector cytokines and/or lineage-defining transcription factors. Here we discuss the critical steps for performing successful multicolor immunophenotyping of mouse T cells in combination with analysis of intracellular molecules after ex vivo isolation.



**Key words** Flow cytometry, Immunophenotyping, Surface marker staining, Intracellular cytokine staining, Intranuclear staining, Cytokine surface capture, Biotinylation, Affinity matrix, Fixation, Permeabilization


## 1 Staining for Cytokines (Cytoplasmic Molecules)

### *1.1 Introduction*

Modern flow cytometers are capable of detecting up to 18 fluorescent parameters and, together with recent advancements in the availability of novel fluorophores, allow for distinguishing evermore functional subgroups of immune cells. However, with the number of parameters also the complexity of an experiment increases tremendously. In order to successfully conduct a 10+ parameter flow cytometry experiment, it is essential to carefully plan the used staining panel to minimize spectral overlap between different channels. Several reviews have been published on how to generate optimized staining panels, and the detailed steps required are beyond the scope of this chapter [1, 2]. However, some of the key points should be mentioned here: First, titration of antibodies is essential to achieve the best possible signal-to-noise ratio. Second, to avoid unspecific staining artifacts it is critical to include a dead-cell marker as well as to perform doublet exclusion (based on area vs. height vs. width gating, e.g., FSC-H vs. FSC-A). Third, it is advisable to construct panels with more than ten parameters by adding only one new marker at a time, which allows spotting


Ari Waisman and Burkhard Becher (eds.), *T-Helper Cells: Methods and Protocols*, Methods in Molecular Biology, vol. 1193,
DOI 10.1007/978-1-4939-1212-4_5, © Springer Science+Business Media New York 2014

problems that arise from spectral overlap before the actual experiment. Fourth, it is essential to have appropriate single-stained compensation controls to set up the flow cytometer [3].

Methods to stain for cytokines have been published already in the early 1990s [4, 5]. These approaches proved to be very useful for the identification and further characterization of different functional subsets within T helper cells, such as Th1, Th2, and Th17 cells and also γδ T cells. Whether these subsets really represent separate lineages is a matter of intense debate [6, 7], but it is evident that the best readout for the function of a given T cell is the cytokine being produced. With the number of measurable parameters increasing, it is possible to detect T cells producing more than one cytokine at a time, and for several disease models these cells have been postulated to be critical [8].

The protocol below describes one approach to perform an intracellular cytokine staining (ICS) with mouse αβ or γδ T cells after ex vivo isolation or after in vitro culture. For the fixation and permeabilization procedure both commercial reagents as well as homemade buffers can be used, which will be described below.

### 1.2 Materials and Reagents

Unless stated otherwise, all staining steps should be performed at 4 °C or on ice to reduce the metabolic activity of the used cells to a minimum. Staining at room temperature will increase unspecific binding of antibodies, and it has been shown that particularly phagocytic cells will still be active at room temperature.

Culture medium: RPMI (Invitrogen) containing 10 % heat-inactivated FCS and Penicillin/Streptomycin (Gibco) and 2 mM L-Glutamine (Gibco).

Phosphate-buffered saline (PBS).

Staining buffer: PBS containing 2 % FBS and 0.01 % $NaN_3$.

Phorbol-12-myristate-13-acetate (PMA) (Applichem).

Ionomycin calcium salt (Applichem).

Dimethyl sulfoxide (DMSO).

Fixable live/dead reagent kit with the desired emission spectrum, for example from Life Technologies (no. L34957) or BioLegend (no. 423102).

Desired surface and intracellular antibodies (depending on the optical setup of your given flow cytometer).

Anti-hamster/rat antibody capture beads (BD, no. 552845).

Cytofix/Cytoperm reagent (BD, no. 554722).

Optional: 4 % formaldehyde solution.

10× Perm/Wash buffer (BD, no. 554723).

Optional: Saponin (Applichem).

Bovine Serum Albumin (BSA) (Applichem).

GolgiPlug containing Brefeldin A (BD, no. 555029) and GolgiStop containing Monensin (BD, no. 554724).

Optional: Brefeldin A.

5 mL polystyrene tubes (12 × 75 mm).

Optional: 96-well V- or U-bottom plates.

Standard flow cytometer capable of detecting the chosen fluorophores (recommended: violet, blue, and red laser lines).

### 1.3 Reagent Preparation

1. Prepare stock solutions of ionomycin and PMA by dilution in DMSO to achieve a concentration of 1 mg/mL for ionomycin and 0.1 mg/mL for PMA and store them at −20 °C.
2. For the Fixable Aqua dead cell stain (Invitrogen), reconstitute one vial of dye with 50 μL of DMSO and store in 5 μL aliquots at −20 °C.
3. If homemade perm/wash buffer is used, prepare PBS containing 0.5 % saponin, 2 % BSA, and 0.01 % $NaN_3$.
4. Prepare restimulation medium: Aliquot the desired volume of culture medium, and add 1:2,000 ionomycin (final concentration 500 ng/mL), 1:2,000 PMA (final concentration 50 ng/mL), and 1:1,000 GolgiPlug or GolgiStop, respectively.
5. For surface staining mix dilute the desired antibodies in staining buffer at 2× the optimal concentration (note that while staining in 5 mL tubes, the residual volume of liquid after decanting will be approximately 50 μL).
6. For the live/dead staining mix dilute the stock solution 1:500 in PBS.
7. For the intracellular staining mix dilute the desired antibodies in perm/wash buffer at 2× the optimal concentration (note that while staining in 5 mL tubes, the residual volume of liquid after decanting will be approximately 50 μL).

### 1.4 Methods

1. Isolate lymphocytes from the organ of interest (see other chapters).
2. After isolation, count the cells. For intracellular stainings it is advisable to start at least with one million of cells, depending on the application and the percentage of T cells in the sample.
3. Transfer the desired number of cells into 5 mL tubes and centrifuge at 400 × $g$ for 5 min at 4 °C. Decant supernatant.
4. Resuspend cells in 1 mL restimulation medium containing ionomycin, PMA, and GolgiPlug. If more than $20 \times 10^6$ cells are being used, scale up the volume accordingly.

5. Incubate the cells for 4–6 h at 37 °C and 5 % $CO_2$.
6. Remove cells from the incubator and centrifuge at 400 × *g* for 5 min at 4 °C, and decant supernatant.
7. Add 4 mL of staining buffer to wash the cells.
8. Centrifuge at 400 × *g* for 5 min at 4 °C, remove supernatant, and drain the tube quickly on a paper towel to remove residual liquid.
9. Add 50 μL of surface staining mix to the cells, and pulse-vortex to mix.
10. Incubate for 20 min at 4 °C, preferably in the dark.
11. Add 1 mL of staining buffer to wash the cells, centrifuge at 400 × *g* for 5 min at 4 °C, remove supernatant, and drain the tube on a paper towel to remove residual liquid.
12. Add 50 μL of live/dead staining mix to the cells, and pulse-vortex to mix.
13. Incubate for 20 min at 4 °C, preferably in the dark.
14. Add 1 mL of staining buffer to wash the cells, centrifuge at 400 × *g* for 5 min at 4 °C, remove supernatant, and drain the tube on a paper towel to remove residual liquid.
15. Add 150 μL of Cytofix/Cytoperm reagent to each tube, and pulse-vortex to mix. Optional: Instead of commercial buffers, formaldehyde can be used for fixation. In this case, resuspend the cells in 100 μL PBS, pulse-vortex to mix, then add 100 μL of 4 % formaldehyde, and pulse-vortex again.
16. Incubate for 20 min at 4 °C, preferably in the dark. Note: After this step, cells can be stored in perm/wash buffer overnight at 4 °C.
17. Add 500 μL of perm/wash to each tube, centrifuge at 400 × *g* for 5 min at 4 °C, remove supernatant, and drain the tube on a paper towel to remove residual liquid. Optional: If homemade perm/wash buffer is used, add 1 mL of homemade perm/wash and incubate for 10 min at room temperature before proceeding to the next step.
18. Add 50 μL of intracellular staining mix (diluted in perm/wash) to the cells, and pulse-vortex to mix.
19. Incubate for 20 min at 4 °C, preferably in the dark.
20. Add 500 μL of perm/wash to each tube, centrifuge at 400 × *g* for 5 min at 4 °C, and remove supernatant. Repeat this washing step once.
21. Resuspend cells in appropriate volume of staining buffer and process samples within 72 h by flow cytometry.
22. Analyze the sample files using a data analysis program or automated data processing algorithms [9].

## 2 Staining for Transcription Factors (Intranuclear Molecules)

### 2.1 Introduction

While the general approach to staining nuclear proteins is identical to the one used to stain cytoplasmic molecules (fix-permeabilize-stain-wash), the location of the target (nucleus vs. cytoplasm) might require a different set of buffers to be used. To assist the investigator, many companies have developed reference tables and protocols that can serve as a starting point in designing the experiment. Depending on the target molecule, different combinations of fixation and permeabilization reagents might be recommended.

The following protocol allows the simultaneous analysis of cell surface molecules and intracellular antigens at the single-cell level. This protocol combines fixation and permeabilization into a single step and does not require continuous exposure to permeabilization buffer for intracellular staining. This protocol is recommended for detecting nuclear antigens such as transcription factors (for example Foxp3) but is also useful for detecting many cytokines.

### 2.2 Materials and Reagents

5 mL polystyrene tubes (12×75 mm).

Directly conjugated antibodies specific for intracellular proteins.

Foxp3 Fixation/Permeabilization Concentrate and Diluent (eBioscience No. 00-5521).

Permeabilization Buffer (10×) (eBioscience No. 00-8333).

### 2.3 Reagent Preparation

1. Prepare fresh Foxp3 Fixation/Permeabilization working solution by diluting Foxp3 Fixation/Permeabilization Concentrate (1 part) with Foxp3 Fixation/Permeabilization Diluent (3 parts). You will need 0.5 mL of the Fixation/Permeabilization working solution for each sample.
2. Prepare a 1× working solution of permeabilization buffer by diluting the 10× concentrate with distilled water prior to use. You will need 4–5 mL of permeabilization buffer for each sample.
3. For surface staining mix dilute the desired antibodies in staining buffer at 2× the optimal concentration (note that while staining in 5 mL tubes, the residual volume of liquid after decanting will be approximately 50 μL).
4. For the live/dead staining mix dilute the stock solution 1:500 in PBS.
5. For the intracellular staining mix dilute the desired antibodies in perm buffer at 2× the optimal concentration (note that while staining in 5 mL tubes, the residual volume of liquid after decanting will be approximately 50 μL).

### 2.4 Methods

1. Isolate lymphocytes from the organ of interest (see other chapters).
2. After isolation, count the cells. For intracellular stainings it is advisable to start at least with one million of cells, depending on the application and the percentage of T cells in the sample.
3. Transfer the desired number of cells into 5 mL tubes and centrifuge at 400 × *g* for 5 min at 4 °C. Decant supernatant.
4. Perform the surface staining as well as staining with a fixable live/dead reagent according to the steps described in Subheading 1.
5. After the last wash, discard the supernatant and pulse-vortex the sample to completely dissociate the pellet.
6. Add 0.5 mL of Foxp3 Fixation/Permeabilization working solution to each tube and pulse-vortex.
7. Incubate at 4 °C for a minimum of 30 min in the dark (murine samples can be incubated for up to 18 h at 4 °C in the dark).
8. Add 2 mL 1× perm buffer to each tube, centrifuge samples at 400 × *g* for 5 min, and then discard the supernatant.
9. Add 50 μL of intracellular staining mix (diluted in perm/wash) to the cells, and pulse-vortex to mix.
10. Incubate in the dark at 4 °C for at least 30 min.
11. Add 2 mL 1× perm buffer to each tube.
12. Centrifuge samples at 400 × *g* for 5 min, and then discard the supernatant.
13. Repeat **steps 13** and **14**.
14. Resuspend stained cells in an appropriate volume of staining buffer and acquire data on a flow cytometer.

## 3 Notes

1. For intracellular staining the viability of the obtained cells is crucial. Hence, it is recommended to process the sample during the previously required isolation steps as fast as possible.
2. As discussed in 2.1, one of the most critical steps for optimal staining is antibody titration. We strongly recommend titrating all antibodies under the experimental conditions, to obtain optimal signal-to-noise ratio. Further information on this topic can be found in ref. 2.
3. Often the FSC-SSC profile of lymphocytes is used to discriminate live from dead cells. However, this is not a definitive criterion, and after fixation and permeabilization of cells even less so.

Therefore, the use of a fixable live/dead reagent is strongly recommended to avoid artifacts from unspecific antibody binding to dead cells. Further information can be found in ref. 10.

4. As stated in the protocol, fixable live/dead reagents need to be diluted in PBS rather than staining buffer since extraneous protein in the buffer will reduce the staining intensity of cells. However, it is possible to add the live/dead reagent directly to the surface staining mix, if this mixture is prepared in PBS. In this case, the preceding washing step needs to be performed using PBS.
5. For restimulation of T cells, PMA and ionomycin are most commonly used. However, given the strong artificial activation induced by these two compounds, it might be beneficial for some assays to use peptides in combination with anti-CD28 for restimulation. This will result in significantly less cytokine production, but will be restricted to the T cells carrying the cognate antigen receptor.
6. Brefeldin A (contained in GolgiPlug) and monensin (contained in GolgiStop) likewise are often used as cytokine secretion inhibitors. However, they have been shown to differentially affect the secretion of a particular cytokine: Monensin, for example, does not inhibit TNFα secretion efficiently. On the other hand, brefeldin A inhibits CD69 surface expression. In our experience, brefeldin A alone is sufficient for most assays, but we recommend testing both compounds for a given experimental setting. Brefeldin A and monensin can also be used simultaneously without negative effects.
7. Commercial buffers for fixation and permeabilization are available from various major manufacturers (BD, eBioscience, BioLegend). However, homemade reagents can be used at comparable efficiency as described in the protocol.
8. A few additional words on nomenclature of fixatives: Probably the most commonly used one is a water solution of formaldehyde ($H_2CO$). However, formalin, formaldehyde, and paraformaldehyde are terms used interchangeably to name the same fixative. Even worse, sometimes an investigator is led to believe that these terms actually denote a different substance.

   At room temperature, *formaldehyde* is a gas. *Formalin* is a formaldehyde dissolved in water. *Paraformaldehyde* is a polymerized form of formaldehyde—it is hardly soluble and cannot be used as a fixative. Saturated solutions of formaldehyde in water, containing 10–15 % methanol as a preservative, are generally called "formaldehyde" and are being sold by most reagent companies. Solutions further diluted (4–10 %) received the name "formalin." When a methanol-free formaldehyde is required, it can be obtained by hydrolysis (depolymerization) of paraformaldehyde. Because of this origin, the methanol-free formaldehyde received (incorrectly) the name "paraformaldehyde." Unfortunately, this incorrect name is still often used in the literature, generating the confusion.

## 4 Part 2: Surface Capture Staining

### 4.1 Summary

While intracellular staining approaches have proven to be useful for the identification of different T cell effector subsets, this technique inevitably kills the analyzed cells. However, for some downstream applications, such as further in vitro culture or adoptive in vivo transfer, it is useful to enrich cells producing a particular cytokine. Unless a genetic mouse model is available, the technique of choice is cell surface capture, which allows for a surface staining of cells producing a given cytokine.

### 4.2 Introduction

Surface capture staining, sometimes also termed "cell-surface affinity matrix technology," is a method for sorting or analyzing cell populations based on the secretion of molecules such as antibodies or cytokines. The first approaches for surface capture staining were developed in the 1990s, and by now several improvements have led to the protocols currently available [11, 12].

The underlying principle is the retention of secreted molecules at the surface of the secreting cell, making them available to conventional surface staining approaches. To do so, a "catch reagent" consisting of an antibody specific for the molecule of interest (e.g., a cytokine) coupled to an antibody binding a ubiquitous surface antigen (e.g., CD45 or CD3) on the target cells is used to stain the cells. During a subsequent incubation period the secreted molecule of interest will be captured by the "catch reagent" on the surface of the cells, followed by conventional surface staining for the molecule of interest.

Comparison to classical intracellular staining approaches has shown that cytokine surface capture staining yields comparable results in terms of cytokine positivity. However, surface capture is more time and reagent consuming and thus only used if viable cells are a requirement for downstream applications. One example of this is adoptive transfer of skewed T helper cells in a setting of autoimmune disease, which allows following the fate of a given T helper lineage without the need for a transgenic mouse model [13].

### 4.3 Materials and Reagents

Unless stated otherwise, all staining steps should be performed at 4 °C or on ice to reduce the metabolic activity of the cells to a minimum.

Culture medium: RPMI (Invitrogen) containing 10 % heat-inactivated FCS and Penicillin/Streptomycin (Gibco) and 2 mM L-Glutamine (Gibco).

Staining buffer: PBS containing 2 % FBS and 0.01 % $NaN_3$.

Phorbol-12-myristate-13-acetate (PMA) (Applichem).

Ionomycin calcium salt (Applichem).

Optional: Peptide antigen of interest.

Optional: Cytokines and neutralizing antibodies for T helper cell skewing: anti-IFN-γ (10 μg/mL; R4-6A2; BioXCell) and anti-IL-12 (10 μg/mL; C17.8; BioXCell) for GM-CSF-secreting cells; anti-IFN-γ, anti-IL-12 (10 μg/mL), IL-2 (10 ng/mL; PeproTech), and IL-4 (50 ng/mL; R&D Systems) for TH2 cells; anti-IFN-γ (10 μg/mL), TGF-β (10 ng/mL; PeproTech), and IL-6 (20 ng/mL; PeproTech) for TH17 cells; and IFN-γ (10 ng/mL; PeproTech) and IL-12 (20 ng/mL; PeproTech) for TH1 cells.

Anti-CD45-Biotin (clone 30F11) or anti-CD3-Biotin (clone 2C11) antibody.

Avidin (Invitrogen, A2667).

Biotin-conjugated anti-cytokine antibodies of choice, e.g., anti-GM-CSF (clone MP1-22E9), anti-IL-17A (clone TC11-18H10), or anti-IFN-γ (clone XMG1.2).

Fluorochrome-conjugated anti-cytokine antibodies of choice, e.g., anti-GM-CSF-PE, anti-IL-17A-APC, anti IFNγ-FITC.

Fluorochrome-conjugated antibodies of choice for surface staining, e.g., anti-CD4-Pacific Blue (clone GK1.5) and anti-CD8-PeCy7 (clone 53.6-7).

Propidium iodide (PI).

Optional: Anti PE-microbeads (Miltenyi).

50 mL tubes.

5 mL polystyrene tubes (12 × 75 mm).

Standard cell sorter capable of detecting the chosen fluorophores.

Optional: AutoMACS (Miltenyi).

### 4.4 Methods

1. Isolate lymphocytes from your organ of interest (see other chapters).
2. Optional: If you want to generate skewed T helper cells, culture them under skewing conditions for Th1, Th2, Th17, or ThGM polarization for 3 days (using anti-CD3 and anti-CD28):
   (a) Th1 cells: IFN-γ (10 ng/mL) and IL-12 (20 ng/mL).
   (b) Th2 cells: Anti-IFN-γ, anti-IL-12 (10 μg/mL), IL-2 (10 ng/mL), and IL-4 (50 ng/mL).
   (c) Th17 cells: Anti-IFN-γ (10 μg/mL), TGF-β (10 ng/mL), and IL-6 (20 ng/mL).

(d) ThGM cells: Anti-IFN-γ (10 μg/mL) and anti-IL-12 (10 μg/mL) (for details see other chapters).

3. Mix the surface capture construct: Dilute anti-CD45 antibody and the respective cytokine antibody in 200 μL of PBS to achieve a final concentration of 1 μg/mL, and add 20 μL of avidin.
4. Incubate for 5 min at RT and vortex again.
5. Resuspend up to $40 \times 10^6$ cells in 200 μL of surface capture construct and incubate for 15 min at 4 °C. It is important to keep the cells cold at this step to prevent secretion of cytokines!
6. Dilute the cells using warm culture medium based on the expected frequency of cytokine-secreting cells as below:
   (a) 1–5 %: $2 \times 10^6$ cells/mL.
   (b) More than 5 %: $1 \times 10^6$ cells/mL.
   (c) 20–50 %: $0.5 \times 10^6$ cells/mL.
7. Incubate cells with ionomycin (final concentration 500 ng/mL) and PMA (final concentration 50 ng/mL) for 3 h at 37 °C and 5 % $CO_2$. Alternatively, peptide and anti-CD28 (final concentration 20 μg/mL) can be used for restimulation, but in this case incubation time might need to be extended.
8. During the incubation phase, keep cells on a slow agitator, or gently mix the cells every 15–30 min to avoid settling.
9. Wash the cells by adding at least the same volume of ice-cold staining buffer, centrifuge at $400 \times g$ for 5 min at 4 °C, and remove supernatant.
10. Add 100 μL of staining mix containing the cytokine detection antibodies as well as surface marker antibodies to the cells, and pulse-vortex to mix.
11. Incubate for 20 min at 4 °C, preferably in the dark.
12. Add 1 mL of staining buffer to wash the cells, centrifuge at $400 \times g$ for 5 min at 4 °C, remove supernatant, and drain the tube on a paper towel to remove residual liquid.
13. Proceed to the cell sorter and sort your cells based on cytokine positivity. Add PI (0.5 μg/mL) prior to starting the sort for exclusion of dead cells.
14. Alternatively, magnetically label the cells using anti-PE microbeads according to the manufacturer's instructions (Miltenyi).

## 5 Notes

1. Similar to intracellular staining approaches, good viability of the used cells is important. Therefore, it is recommended to process the sample during the prior isolation steps as fast as possible.

2. The most critical point in the surface capture assay is the prevention of neighboring cells catching the secreted cytokine, which will lead to false-positive events. In order to avoid this, the cell suspension must not be too dense during the cytokine secretion phase; that is, it should not exceed $5 \times 10^6$ cells/mL. Furthermore, if the total amount of cytokine in the medium starts to rise above a certain level, all cells will be able to catch the cytokine. However, during flow cytometric analysis this problem can be spotted by a shift in fluorescence of the total cell population.
3. Several major manufacturers offer kits that include ready-to-use catch reagents optimized for some experimental settings. We recommend evaluating these kits on an individual experimental basis.
4. As mentioned in the protocol, instead of an electronic cell sorter, a magnetic cell sorting approach can be utilized. In this case, the anti-cytokine antibody needs to be labeled with PE in order to use anti-PE microbeads for the subsequent isolation steps. Further information on this approach can be obtained from the manufacturer (Miltenyi).

## References


1. Perfetto SP, Chattopadhyay PK, Roederer M (2004) Seventeen-colour flow cytometry: unravelling the immune system. Nat Rev Immunol 4:648–655
2. Mahnke YD, Roederer M (2007) Optimizing a multicolor immunophenotyping assay. Clin Lab Med 27:469–485, v
3. Roederer M (2001) Spectral compensation for flow cytometry: visualization artifacts, limitations, and caveats. Cytometry 45:194–205
4. Sander B, Andersson J, Andersson U (1991) Assessment of cytokines by immunofluorescence and the paraformaldehyde-saponin procedure. Immunol Rev 119:65–93
5. Jung T, Schauer U, Heusser C, Neumann C, Rieger C (1993) Detection of intracellular cytokines by flow cytometry. J Immunol Methods 159:197–207
6. Bluestone JA, Mackay CR, O'Shea JJ, Stockinger B (2009) The functional plasticity of T cell subsets. Nat Rev Immunol 9:811–816
7. Zhu J, Yamane H, Paul WE (2010) Differentiation of effector CD4 T cell populations *. Annu Rev Immunol 28:445–489
8. Hirota K et al (2011) Fate mapping of IL-17-producing T cells in inflammatory responses. Nat Immunol 12:255–263
9. Aghaeepour N et al (2013) Critical assessment of automated flow cytometry data analysis techniques. Nat Meth 10:228–238
10. Perfetto SP et al. (2010) Amine-reactive dyes for dead cell discrimination in fixed samples. Curr Protoc Cytom Chapter 9, Unit 9.34
11. Brosterhus H et al (1999) Enrichment and detection of live antigen-specific CD4(+) and CD8(+) T cells based on cytokine secretion. Eur J Immunol 29:4053–4059
12. Manz R, Assenmacher M, Pflüger E, Miltenyi S, Radbruch A (1995) Analysis and sorting of live cells according to secreted molecules, relocated to a cell-surface affinity matrix. Proc Natl Acad Sci U S A 92: 1921–1925
13. Codarri L et al (2011) RORγt drives production of the cytokine GM-CSF in helper T cells, which is essential for the effector phase of autoimmune neuroinflammation. Nat Immunol 12:560–567

# Chapter 6

# Tracking Cells and Monitoring Proliferation


## Vinko Tosevski and Florian Mair



## Abstract

In many areas of immunology it is desirable to be able to track particular cells throughout an assay, whether it be in vivo or in vitro. There are two classes or reagents used for this purpose—general protein labels (reactive compounds that form random covalent bonds with amino groups on cellular proteins) and general membrane labels (lipophilic compounds that partition stably but non-covalently into the plasma membrane). The fluorescein derivative, carboxyfluorescein diacetate succinimidyl ester, CFDA-SE (general protein label), has been found to be particularly well suited for the purpose of cell tracking. Once labeled, cells can be tracked both in vivo and in vitro. Moreover, due to the randomness of the labeling, cells undergoing division maintain half of the staining intensity of the parent cell. This halving of the staining intensity additionally allows for monitoring of cells undergoing division for 6–8 consecutive cycles.



**Key words** CFSE, CFDA-SE, Cell proliferation, Cell tracking, Cell migration, Differentiation, Kinetics, Immune response, Division modeling, Dye dilution


## 1 Introduction

Weston and Parish were the first to report using CFDA-SE for long-term tracking of lymphocyte migration [1]. Few years later, their colleague Bruce Lyons noticed that the intracellular fluorescent label is divided equally between daughter cells upon cell division, resulting in a sequential halving of fluorescence. The technique was applicable to in vitro cell division, as well as in vivo division of adoptively transferred cells, and could resolve multiple successive generations using flow cytometry [2]. Indeed, the tracking of lymphocyte division using CFDA-SE has become a routine procedure in many laboratories since its first description in 1994. In particular, the procedure has been used for the analysis of cell division in vivo in mice and in vitro using mouse and human lymphocytes. CFDA-SE has the additional advantage that it can be used to track lymphocyte migration and positioning within tissues and lymphoid organs [2]. In fact, the dye was originally developed for this purpose, being stably incorporated into lymphocytes and allowing the


Ari Waisman and Burkhard Becher (eds.), *T-Helper Cells: Methods and Protocols*, Methods in Molecular Biology, vol. 1193, DOI 10.1007/978-1-4939-1212-4_6, © Springer Science+Business Media New York 2014

tracking of lymphocytes in vivo for many months [1]. CFSE-labeled cells have also been used for in vivo and in vitro cytotoxicity assays [3–6].

Carboxyfluorescein diacetate succinimidyl ester is often referred to incorrectly in the literature as "CFSE"—it should NOT be confused with carboxyfluorescein succinimidyl ester (CFSE), which is not the diacetate form and is not cell permeable. Although the CFSE is only an intermediate molecular species in the process of cell labeling, we will, nevertheless, refer to the whole assay as CFSE assay.

A colorless nonpolar derivative of fluorescein, CFDA-SE diffuses into the cytoplasm where its acetate substituents are cleaved by nonspecific esterases, forming the fluorescent product carboxyfluorescein succinimidyl ester (CFSE). CFSE reacts with amine groups on peptides and proteins under physiologic conditions, forming a stable amide bond. The reaction releases *N*-hydroxysuccinimide and results in a fluorescein molecule bound to a protein.

Extremely bright labeling is readily achieved due to trapping of the polar CFSE within the cytoplasm, making it possible to detect six to eight rounds of cell division so long as labeling levels used do not alter protein regions critical for cell function.

## 2 Material and Reagents

CFSE is available from the Molecular Probes division of Invitrogen (Carlsbad, CA), Sigma-Aldrich (St. Louis, MO), and a variety of other suppliers.

### 2.1 Reagent Preparation

CFDA-SE is prepared at a stock concentration 1,000-fold higher than the final usage concentration (for example, 2 mM if the final concentration is 2 μM) in anhydrous DMSO. Aliquot into single-usage vials and store at −20 °C. CFDA-SE will hydrolyze quickly at room temperature in the presence of water, and much more slowly at −20 °C. If your cells show decreased labeling with the same stock of CFDA-SE, hydrolysis is the likely cause.

## 3 Method

1. Suspend your cells in PBS or HBSS containing 0.1 % BSA. Cell concentrations can range widely from $1 \times 10^6$ cells/mL (for in vitro experiments) up to $5 \times 10^7$ cells/mL (for adoptive transfer). The cells should be in single-cell suspension—if necessary, filter them through nylon mesh immediately prior to labeling. Total reaction volumes should not exceed 4 mL in

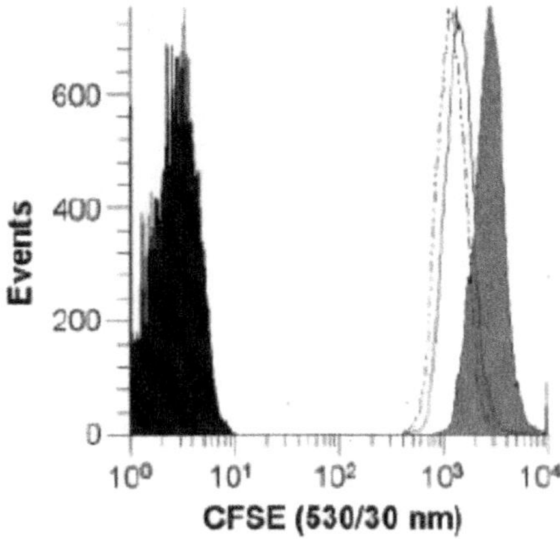


**Fig. 1** Stability of CFDA-SE staining intensity during the first 48 h of culture (*adapted from* [6]). Peripheral blood mononuclear cells were stained with the CFDA-SE and cultured at 37 °C in complete medium without stimulus. Samples were collected immediately after staining (*filled gray histograms*) or after 24 h (*unfilled histogram, continuous line*) or 48 h (*unfilled histogram, dotted line*), fixed, and analyzed. Note that day 1, not day 0, would represent the starting point for a dye dilution study

a 15 mL tube, so prepare cell suspensions at no greater than 2 mL each.

2. Prepare a solution of CFDA-SE from your DMSO stock in PBS/0.1 % BSA at 2× the final labeling concentration; if you are labeling at 5 μM, prepare a 10 μM solution. Prepare a volume of CFDA-SE equal to your cell volume above (no more than 2 mL per labeling reaction).
3. Add an equal volume of CFDA-SE solution to your cell suspension. Mix gently and incubate for 10 min at 37 °C.
4. Immediately fill the labeling tube to the top with the tissue culture media intended for culture (such as RPMI/10 % FCS) and centrifuge. Wash the cells three times with tissue culture media.

Although cells are considered stained at this point, their initial intensity does not represent the starting point for a proliferation assay since a substantial fraction of total dye is lost during the first 24 h (*see* Fig. 1), as the cells clear damaged or short-lived proteins and those destined for export. Also, one cannot simply assume that dye concentration(s) reported in the literature will work for every cell type or experimental setting. Rather, they must be tested and modified as necessary to assure that, after 24 h in culture, labeled cells exhibit high viability, unaltered function, and bright homogeneous staining.

## 4 Notes

Cells are usually labeled at a final CFDA-SE concentration of 0.5–5 μM. The literature reports concentrations ranging from 0.2 to 10 μM and even higher. For best results, do a titration and find the lowest concentration of CFDA-SE that will give effective cell labeling—this will vary from cell type to cell type, and also with the application. CFDA-SE labeling is somewhat toxic and can induce growth arrest and apoptosis in some cell types—therefore, it is important to find the lowest acceptable labeling concentration and check the viability after labeling. As a rough guide, 0.5–2 μM is usually enough for in vitro experiments—cell tracking and generational analysis in transplanted cells may require 2–5 μM. Incubation time is usually from 5 to 10 min—again, titrate to find the minimal effective conditions. We usually label in PBS containing 0.1 % BSA. All post-labeling washes should be carried out in complete media (such as RPMI with 10 % FCS)—your intended tissue culture media is ideal. The high protein concentration inactivates unreacted CFDA-SE.

### References


1. Weston SA, Parish CR (1990) New fluorescent dyes for lymphocyte migration studies. Analysis by flow cytometry and fluorescence microscopy. J Immunol Methods 133:87–97
2. Lyons AB, Parish CR (1994) Determination of lymphocyte division by flow cytometry. J Immunol Methods 171:131–137
3. Wells AD, Gudmundsdottir H, Turka LA (1997) Following the fate of individual T cells throughout activation and clonal expansion. Signals from T cell receptor and CD28 differentially regulate the induction and duration of a proliferative response. J Clin Invest 100:3173–3183
4. Bird JJ et al (1998) Helper T cell differentiation is controlled by the cell cycle. Immunity 9:229–237
5. Li Y et al (1999) Blocking both signal 1 and signal 2 of T-cell activation prevents apoptosis of alloreactive T cells and induction of peripheral allograft tolerance. Nat Med 5:1298–1302
6. Gett AV, Hodgkin PD (2000) A cellular calculus for signal integration by T cells. Nat Immunol 1: 239–244

# Chapter 7

# Mass Cytometry Analysis of Human T Cell Phenotype and Function

**Evan W. Newell and Lai Li Yun**

## Abstract

Mass cytometry is a form of flow cytometry based on single-cell mass spectrometry that uses monoisotopic elemental labels to probe individual cells. Reduced cross talk between channels and an ability to measure >30 independent cellular parameters make this an attractive approach for high-dimensional analysis of cellular phenotypes and function. Here, methods of using this approach for the analysis of human T cell surface markers and intracellular cytokines are described.

**Key words** Mass cytometry, Cytometry by time-of-flight (CyTOF), Flow cytometry, Intracellular cytokine staining

## 1 Introduction

Mass cytometry (also known as cytometry by time-of-flight, CyTOF™) is a single-cell mass spectrometry-based flow cytometry method that uses isotopically purified heavy metal elements as tags and allows analysis of >30 cellular markers per cell with many more possible [1]. The technical benefits of mass cytometry are clear. In addition to the large number of parameters used, there is greatly reduced cross talk between channel greatly simplifying analysis and interpretation of the data. This approach has allowed for the simultaneous assessment of cytokine responses in a broad range of cell types with a large number of intracellular signaling molecules [2]. The power of this approach has been greatly extended by the use of cellular barcoding technology, originally developed for fluorescence flow cytometry [3], allowing the simultaneous analysis of a large number of stimulation conditions in a single cytometry sample [4]. It has also been used to investigate the relationship between T cell antigen specificity, surface marker phenotypes, and the broad range of combinatorial functional capacities that human $CD8^+$ T cells can express [5–7]. Here, updated methods for the analysis

Ari Waisman and Burkhard Becher (eds.), *T-Helper Cells: Methods and Protocols*, Methods in Molecular Biology, vol. 1193, DOI 10.1007/978-1-4939-1212-4_7, © Springer Science+Business Media New York 2014

of T cell phenotype and function in human peripheral blood mononuclear cells are described.

To assess the mostly unperturbed phenotypic profiles in parallel with the functional capacities of human T lymphocytes, short-duration (3 h) stimulation with either PMA+ionomycin or anti-CD3 (+/− anti-CD28) is used. During this short time frame, minimal changes to surface marker expression levels are observed. One exception is the cleavage and release of CD62L (and CD16 from NK cells). To prevent this, a metalloproteinase inhibitor (TAPI-2) is included in the stimulation medium to block this cleavage with no known nonspecific effects [8]. To trap all possible intracellular cytokines and chemokines that are produced during stimulation, a combination of brefeldin A and monensin is added at the time of stimulation used to block secretion. A consequence is that induced surface expression of CD69 is also blocked. Therefore, CD69 can be probed intracellularly. However, unlike a previously available clone (MCA1442 AbDSerotec), to our knowledge the only CD69 antibody currently available (FN50 clone) does not work well as an intracellular stain of fixed cells. Thus, CD69 used as a surface marker can identify previously activated cells or tissue-resident T cells that express CD69 prior to stimulation. To probe for cytotoxic granule release activity, metal-labeled anti-CD107a is included in the stimulation medium, which binds to the intravesicular CD107a that is transiently exposed during cytotoxic granule secretion [9]. The cellular surface marker and intracellular cytokine antibodies and clone names used for these experiments are listed in Subheading 3.3. In addition to intracellular cytokines, granzyme B, perforin, CD40L, and CTLA-4 are probed intracellularly. Expression of CD40L and/or CTLA-4 is induced on some T cells upon stimulation and these proteins are also trapped intracellularly by brefeldin A and/or monensin. Lastly, a new method for identifying dead cells with cisplatin will be used in conjunction with this method [10]. Altogether, this method has been developed with the goal of maximizing the number of phenotypic and functional markers that can be assessed simultaneously on T cells and it is amenable for use with alternate applications.

## 2 Materials

For all reagents, it is important to avoid heavy metal contamination, which can be detected by the mass cytometer. In particular, detergents used to clean glass can contain barium, which can be incorporated into cells and detected during analysis. This contamination is very difficult to remove from glass after it has been washed. Thus, as a general rule, all buffers should be prepared and stored in disposable plastic containers (or dedicated glass containers that have not come in contact with dish-washing detergent). Also, in general, all buffers are stored refrigerated at 4 °C.

1. $dH_2O$: milliQ deionized water directly from the milliQ tap or stored in a disposable plastic container.
2. Antibody conjugation kits: DVS sciences DN3 antibody conjugation kits containing W-, R-, and L-buffers, lyophilized DN3 polymers, lanthanide chloride stock solutions.
3. Metal chloride stock solutions: If not provided by DVS Sciences, Inc., monoisotopic metal-chloride salts dissolved in DVS L-buffer. Isotopes purchased from Trace Scientific include the following: Gd-155, Gd-157, Dy-161, Dy-163 and Yb-173 chloride salts.
4. 0.5 mL 30 kDa concentrator: Millipore UFC503096 (50 kDa also ok).
5. 0.5 mL 3 kDa concentrator: Millipore UFC500396.
6. 0.5 M tris(2-carboxyethyl) phosphine (TCEP) solution: Pierce Cat. #77720.
7. Antibody stabilizer buffer: Candor-Bioscience CAN131125.
8. Phosphate-buffered saline (PBS): Purchased from Gibco® Cat. #10010031.
9. Complete RPMI: RPMI 1640 (Gibco® Cat. #11875119) supplemented with 10 % fetal bovine serum (FBS, Gibco® Cat. #16140071), Glutamine/penicillin/streptomycin (Gibco® Cat. #10378016), 55 μM 2-mercapto-ethanol (Gibco® Cat. #21985023), and 10 mM HEPES (Gibco® Cat. # 15630080).
10. 96-Well flat-bottom high protein-binding plates: NUNC Cat. #NUNC 442404.
11. 96-Well round-bottom plates: NUNC Cat. #NUNC 163320.
12. PMA + ionomycin stock solutions 500× stock solution: 75 μg/mL Phorbol 12-myristate 13-acetate (PMA) (Sigma Cat. #P1585) and 500 μM Ionomycin (Sigma Cat. #I0634) dissolved in DMSO aliquoted and frozen at −20 °C.
13. 1,000× brefeldin A (eBioscience Cat. #00-4506-51) stored at 4 °C.
14. 1,000× monensin (Biolegend Cat. # 420701) stored at 4 °C.
15. TAPI-2 10 mM (100×) stock solution: 10 mM TAPI-2 (BioVision Cat. #2069-1) dissolved in $dH_2O$ aliquoted and frozen at −20 °C.
16. 0.5 mL 0.1 μm spin filters: Millipore Cat. #UFC30VV00.
17. Stimulatory anti-CD3 and anti-CD28 antibodies: Anti-CD3 clone: OKT3 anti-CD28 clone: CD28.2, low endotoxin azide free format, Biolegend.
18. Cytometry buffer (CB): PBS containing 4 % fetal calf serum (or 0.2 % bovine serum albumin), 2 mM EDTA (pH 8.0) (First Base Cat. #BUF-1052), and 0.05 % sodium azide. Filter and store refrigerated at 4 °C.

19. 2 % Paraformaldehyde (PFA) fixative buffer: Made fresh from 16 % stock solution (Electron Microscopy Sciences Cat. #15710) aliquoted and frozen at −80 °C. Dilute to 2 % PFA in PBS (e.g., add 125 μL of 16 % PFA to 875 μL of PBS) immediately before use.
20. Cisplatin: 100 mM stock solution of cisplatin (Sigma Cat. #479306) in $dH_2O$ aliquoted and frozen at −80 °C. Dilute to 200 μM in ice-cold PBS immediately prior to use.
21. Fix/Ir-Interchelator solution: 1 mL 2 % PFA + 1:2,000 Ir-Interchelator (DVS Sciences, Inc.) in PBS.
22. Permeabilization buffer (PB): 1× permeabilization buffer diluted from the purchased 10× stock solution (Biolegend Cat. #421002) using milliQ deionized water.
23. Stimulation +/− PMA + ionomycin (150 ng/mL PMA, 1 μM ionomycin; make 500× stock of both combined frozen at −20 °C).

## 3 Methods

### 3.1 Antibody Conjugation Protocol

This protocol is very similar to an early protocol suggested by DVS Sciences, Inc. More recent DVS protocols should also work (*see* **Note 1**).

1. Spin DN3 polymer tubes for 10 s to ensure that reagent is at the bottom of the tube.
2. Label tubes and add 95 μL of L buffer to each tube.
3. Add 5 μL metal (if stock is 100 mM add 2.5 μL).
4. Vortex to mix and incubate in 37 °C water bath for 1 h.
5. Prepare Abs:
   (a) Using 30 kDa concentrator, take 100 μg of antibody and add R-buffer up to 500 μL total.
   (b) Spin tubes for 5 min @ 4 °C, discard flow-through, add 450 μL R-buffer, and spin once more.
   (c) During centrifugation, dilute 0.5 M TCEP stock to 6 mM in R-buffer (12 μL 0.5 M TCEP, add to 1 mL R-buffer).
   (d) Discard flow-through and add 100 μL of 6 mM TCEP to each antibody.
   (e) Incubate at 37 °C water bath for 30 min (do not exceed).
6. Transfer the 100 μL of metal + polymer to 3 kDa spin filter, add 150 μL L-buffer to polymer PCR tube to wash, add to metal, and spin for 25 min @ 4 °C.
7. For the antibody, add 350 μL C-buffer after 30-min incubation to filter and spin for 5 min @ 4 °C.

8. Discard flow-through, spin with 450 μL W-buffer for 5 min, and repeat once.
9. Discard flow-through, add 150 μL W-buffer to Ab, transfer, and mix with metal + polymer in 3 kDa filter.
10. Mix and spin for 10 min and leave overnight at RT.
11. Next day, add 450 μL W-buffer to 3 kDa filter and transfer to a new 30 kDa filter. Spin for 5 min.
12. Discard flow-through, add 450 μL W-buffer, and spin for 5 min. Discard flow-through and repeat 4×.
13. Add 100 μL W-buffer, mix, and transfer to a fresh low-protein-binding Eppendorf tube.
14. Measure concentration by Nanodrop (Protein A280).
15. Add 100 μL of antibody stabilizer for each conjugated antibody. Calculate the final concentration by the formula (accounting for the estimated concentrator dead volume of 50 μL, absorbance measured in 150 μL volume, and final volume of 250 μL with antibody stabilizer) absorbance/1.4 × 600 μg/mL.

### 3.2 Cell Preparation and Stimulation

1. Human peripheral blood mononuclear cells (PBMC) are isolated by Ficoll gradient using previously established standard procedures [11], cryopreserved, and thawed before use, as described [12].
2. If using anti-CD3 +/− anti-CD28 for stimulation: Prepare 96-well flat-bottom plate for stimulation by adding 100 μL of PBS containing 1 μg/mL anti-CD3 ±5 μg/mL anti-CD28. Store at 4 °C overnight and wash the next day 3× with complete RPMI before adding cells (**step 5**). If antibody stimulation is not used, round-bottom 96-well plates can be used.
3. After thawing, wash cells in complete RPMI, and culture overnight at 37 °C at ~10 million/mL and 1 mL/well of a 24-well flat-bottom plate.
4. Harvest cells from the 24-well plate by pipetting up and down, count, spin down, and resuspend at high concentration for the next step (for $1–3 \times 10^6$ cells per condition).
5. In each well with a final volume of 100 μL add 1–3 × 10 cells + 1× brefeldin A + 1× monensin + 1× TAPI-2 + 2.5 μg/mL Eu-153 metal-conjugated anti-CD107a (filter before use) ±1× PMA + ionomycin. This can be achieved by mixing 50 μL of cells (at $20–60 \times 10^6$/mL) with 25 μL of 4× diluted TAPI-2 + brefeldin A + monensin + anti-CD107a (filtered with 0.1 μm spin filter) and 25 μL of complete RPMI or complete RPMI containing 4× PMA + ionomycin.
6. Incubate cells at 37 °C for 3 h. At the end of this incubation, add 100 μL ice-cold CB buffer. If using flat-bottom plates,

harvest by vigorously pipetting up and down and transfer to 96-well round-bottom plate. Proceed to Subheading 3.3 for cell staining.

### 3.3 Mass Cytometry Staining Cocktail Preparation

Make each antibody cocktail on the day of use. Optimal concentrations of each antibody can be determined by titration experiments; 1–10 μg/mL final concentrations of each antibody are normally used. For each antibody cocktail containing metal-conjugated antibodies, filtering the antibodies with a 0.1 μm spin filter may reduce spurious signal from antibody aggregated. Centrifuging each antibody stock at high speed before use and avoiding the bottom of these tubes when taking antibodies from the antibody stocks may also reduce antibody aggregates.

1. *Primary surface staining cocktail*: Make enough for 50 μL per sample in CB.
   (a) PE-anti-γδTCR 1:25 (Invitrogen, Cat. # MHGD04, Clone: SA6.E9) (*see* **Note 2**).
   (b) APC-anti-CD161 1:25 (Miltenyi, Cat. #130-092-678, Clone: 191B8).
2. *Secondary surface staining cocktail*: Make enough for 50 μL per sample and filter before use in CB.
   (a) Anti-CD14 Qdot 800 1:200 (Invitrogen, Cat. #Q10064 Clone: TüK4). Quantum dots contain cadmium and can be detected by the mass cytometer at atomic masses 112 and 114.
   (b) Ln-115 conjugated anti-CD57 ~1 μg/mL (Biolegend, Clone: HCD57).
   (c) La-139 conjugated anti-CD45 ~5 μg/mL (Biolegend, Clone: HI30).
   (d) Ce*-140 conjugated anti-CD5 ~10 μg/mL (Biolegend, Clone: UCHT2) (**see* **Note 3**).
   (e) Nd-142 conjugated anti-HLA-DR ~5 μg/mL (Biolegend, Clone: L243).
   (f) Nd-143 conjugated anti-CD62L ~5 μg/mL (BD, Clone: DREG-56).
   (g) Nd-145 conjugated anti-CD16 ~5 μg/mL (Biolegend, Clone: 3G8).
   (h) Nd-146 conjugated anti-CD8 ~5 μg/mL (Biolegend, Clone: SK1).
   (i) Nd-148 conjugated anti-CD85j ~5 μg/mL (R&D Systems, Clone: TS2/16).
   (j) Sm-149 conjugated anti-CD4 ~5 μg/mL (Biolegend, Clone: SK3).

(k) Eu-151 conjugated anti-CD27 ~5 μg/mL (eBioscience, Clone: LG.7F9).

(l) Sm-152 conjugated anti-CD45RO ~5 μg/mL (Biolegend, Clone: UCHL1).

(m) Eu-154 conjugated anti-CD3 ~5 μg/mL (Biolegend, Clone: UCHT-1).

(n) Gd-156 conjugated anti-CD19 ~5 μg/mL (Biolegend, Clone: H1B19).

(o) Gd-157* conjugated anti-CXCR3 ~10 μg/mL (Biolegend, Clone: G025H7).

(p) Gd-158 conjugated anti-CD56 ~3 μg/mL (BD, Clone: NCAM16.2).

(q) Tb-159 streptavidin ~2 μg/mL recombinant protein (*see* **Note 4**).

(r) Gd-160 conjugated anti-CD28 ~5 μg/mL (Biolegend, Clone: CD28.2).

(s) Dy-161* conjugated anti-CD38 ~5 μg/mL (Biolegend, Clone: HIT2).

(t) Dy-163* conjugated anit-CD127 ~5 μg/mL (Biolegend, Clone: A019D5).

(u) Ho-165 conjugated anti-Va7.2 ~5 μg/mL (Biolegend, Clone: 3C10).

(v) Er-167 conjugated anti-PE ~5 μg/mL (Biolegend, Clone: PE001).

(w) Er-168 conjugated anti-CCR7 ~5 μg/mL (R&D, Clone: 150503).

(x) Tm-169 conjugated anti-CCR5 ~10 μg/mL (Biolegend, Clone: HEK/1/85a).

(y) Er-170 conjugated anti-APC ~5 μg/mL (Biolegend, Clone: APC003).

(z) Yb-174 conjugated anti-CD45RA ~5 μg/mL (eBioscience, Clone: JS-83).

(aa) Yb-176 conjugated anti-CXCR5 ~10 μg/mL (BD, Clone: RF8B2).

3. *Primary intracellular staining cocktail*: Make enough for 50 μL per sample in PB.

   (a) Biotinylated anti-IL-10 ~5 μg/mL.

4. *Secondary intracellular staining cocktail*: Make enough for 50 μL per sample in PB and filter before use.

   (a) Pr-141 conjugated anti-IFN-γ ~5 μg/mL (eBiosciene, Clone: 4S.B3).

   (b) Sm-147 conjugated anti-TNF-a ~2 μg/mL (eBiosciene, Clone: Mab11).

(c) Nd-150 conjugated anti-Granzyme B ~2 μg/mL (Abcam, Clone: CLB-GB11).

(d) Gd-155* conjugated anti-CTLA-4 ~5 μg/mL (BD, Clone: BNI3).

(e) Dy-162* conjugated anti-IL-4 ~5 μg/mL (Biolegend, Clone: MP4-25D2).

(f) Dy-164 conjugated anti-IL-17 ~5 μg/mL (Biolegend, Clone: BL168).

(g) Er-166 conjugated anti-IL-2 ~3 μg/mL (eBioscience, Clone: MQ1-17H12).

(h) Yb-171 conjugated anti-CD40L ~5 μg/mL (eBioscience, Clone: 24-31).

(i) Yb-172 conjugated anti-GM-CSF ~5 μg/mL (Biolegend, Clone: BVD2-21C11).

(j) Yb-173* conjugated anti-perforin ~5 μg/mL (Abcam, Clone: B-D48).

(k) Lu-175 conjugated anti-MIP-1beta ~3 μg/mL (BD, Clone: D21-1351).

### 3.4 Mass Cytometry Staining Protocol

1. In 96-well round-bottom plates, 1–3 million cells per well should be used.
2. From Subheading 3.2, cells should be resuspended in a mixture of complete RPMI and CB and pellet cells by centrifugation and remove supernatant (*see* **Note 5**).
3. Resuspend in 100 μL of 200 μM cisplatin in ice-cold PBS.
4. Incubate plates on ice for 5 min.
5. Add 100 μL CB to quench, pellet cells, and remove supernatant.
6. Resuspend cells in 50 μL of primary antibody *primary surface staining cocktail.*
7. Ice for 30 min.
8. Fill with CB to 200 μL, pellet cells, and remove supernatant.
9. Fill with CB, pellet cells, and remove supernatant.
10. Resuspend carefully in 50 μL *secondary surface staining cocktail.*
11. Incubate for 30 min on ice.
12. Top up with CB buffer to 200 μL (add 150 μL), pellet cells, and remove supernatant.
13. Fill with CB, pellet cells, and remove supernatant.
14. Fill with PBS, pellet cells, and remove supernatant.
15. Resuspend well in 150 μL of 2 % PFA in PBS.
16. Seal plate and store/incubate at 4 °C overnight (or longer—several days to weeks appears not to be a problem).

*Day 2, Intracellular Staining*

1. Add 50 μL PB, pellet cells, and remove supernatant.
2. Fill with PB, pellet cells, and remove supernatant.
3. Resuspend in 50 μL *primary intracellular staining cocktail.*
4. Fill with PB, pellet cells, and remove supernatant.
5. Fill with PB, pellet cells, and remove supernatant.
6. Resuspend in 50 μL *secondary intracellular staining cocktail.*
7. Fill with PB, pellet cells, and remove supernatant.
8. Fill with PB, pellet cells, and remove supernatant.
9. Fill with cold CB, pellet cells, and remove supernatant.
10. Fill with cold CB, pellet cells, and remove supernatant.
11. Resuspend in freshly thawed 2 % PFA + 1:2,000 Ir-Interchelator in PBS (100 μL/well).
12. Incubate for 20 min at room temp.
13. Top up with PBS to 200 μL, pellet cells, and remove supernatant.
14. Fill with CB, pellet cells, and remove supernatant.
15. Fill with $dH_2O$, pellet cells, and remove supernatant.
16. Fill with $dH_2O$, pellet cells, and remove supernatant (*see* **Note 6**).
17. Resuspend in $dH_2O$ and filter with 30 μm mesh for running on CyTOF.

### 3.5 Data Analysis

1. Basic considerations of mass cytometer setup, usage, and tuning have been well described [13]. Use DVS acquisition software to create .fcs files for subsequent analysis.
2. Mass cytometry .fcs files can be used with a variety of cytometry analysis software packages including FlowJo, Cytobank, and DVS-Cytobank. For the example analysis shown here (*see* Fig. 1) FlowJo software is used. Care must be taken to ensure that the bioexponential (logicle) transform used by FlowJo software is set up correctly. That is, appropriate "top-of-scale" and "w" values must be chosen. Also, it is important that all parameters except time and "cell length" are fixed for all parameters and samples being compared.
3. Standard flow cytometry analysis software can be used to check that each antibody is performing well. Knowledge of the expected staining pattern for each antibody being used is important for this validation. Side-by-side comparison with fluorescence flow cytometry can also be used to validate staining (*see* **Notes 7** and **8**).

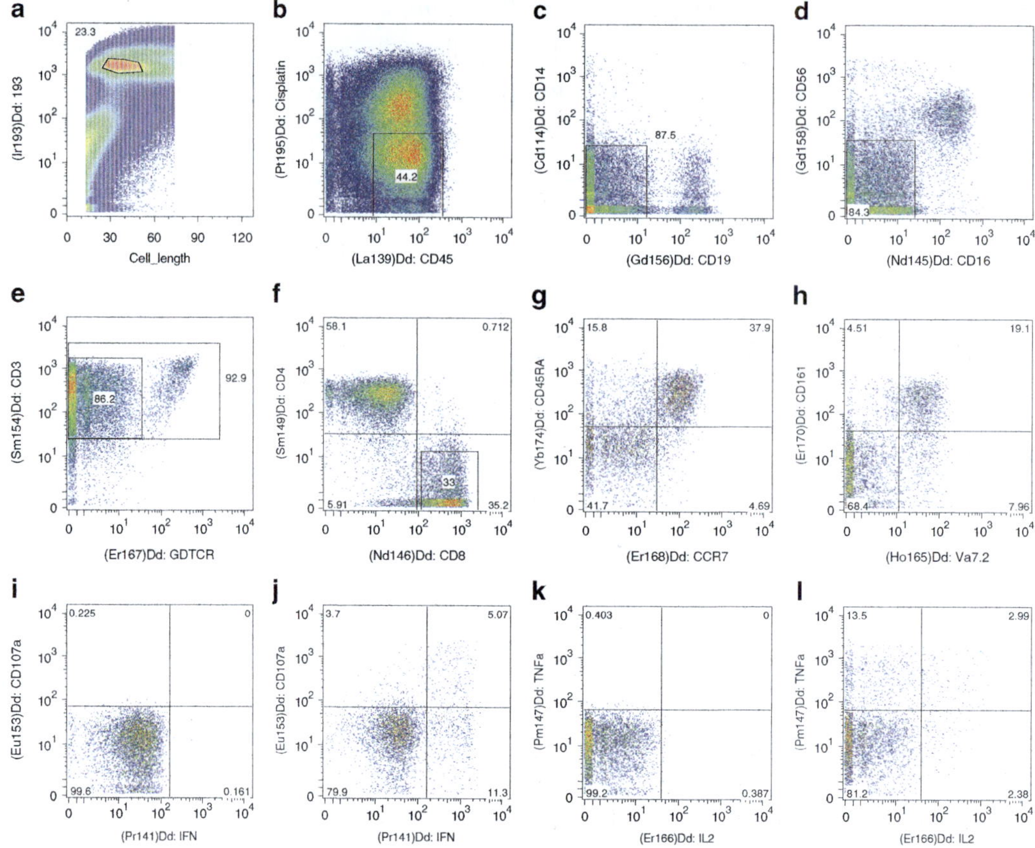


**Fig. 1** Example mass cytometry analysis of human peripheral blood T cells. (**a**) Events are first gated based on DNA content and "cell length" to identify single cells. (**b**) Next, live (cisplatin-negative), $CD45^+$ hematopoietic cells are chosen before isolated T cells by gating on (**c**) $CD14^-CD19^-$, (**d**) $CD56^-CD16^-$, and (**e**) $CD3^+$ cells (larger gate represents total T cells used for analysis shown in Fig. 2). (**f**) $\gamma\delta$TCR-negative cells identified in the smaller gate cells are then further segregated by CD4 and CD8. (**g**) CD45RA vs. CCR7 expression phenotypes are shown for $CD8^+$ T cells. (**h**) Further analyzing $CD8^+$ T cells, the expression of CD161 and V$\alpha$7.2 is shown as a way to identify $CD161^+V\alpha7.2^+$ mucosa-associated invariant T (MAIT) cells. To assess the functional capacities of these $CD4^-CD8^+$ T cells, the cytokine expression of (**i**, **k**) unstimulated cells is compared with (**j**, **l**) PMA + ionomycin-stimulated cells. (**i**, **j**) Stimulation-induced degranulation and exposure of CD107a are shown together with the induction of IFN-gamma expression. (**k**, **l**) Stimulation-induced expression of IL-2 and TNF-a is also shown

4. There is no correct way to analyze high-dimensional cellular data. Various forms of clustering algorithms or principal component analysis have been used to make better sense of the high-dimensional data produced using mass cytometry [2, 4, 5, 7]. The Spanning-tree Progression Analysis of Density-normalized Events (SPADE) [14, 15] algorithm is particularly useful because it has been developed specifically for this purpose, allows quick visualization of general patterns in the data, and is complementary to other methods (*see* Fig. 2 for example output using this algorithm with this data produced

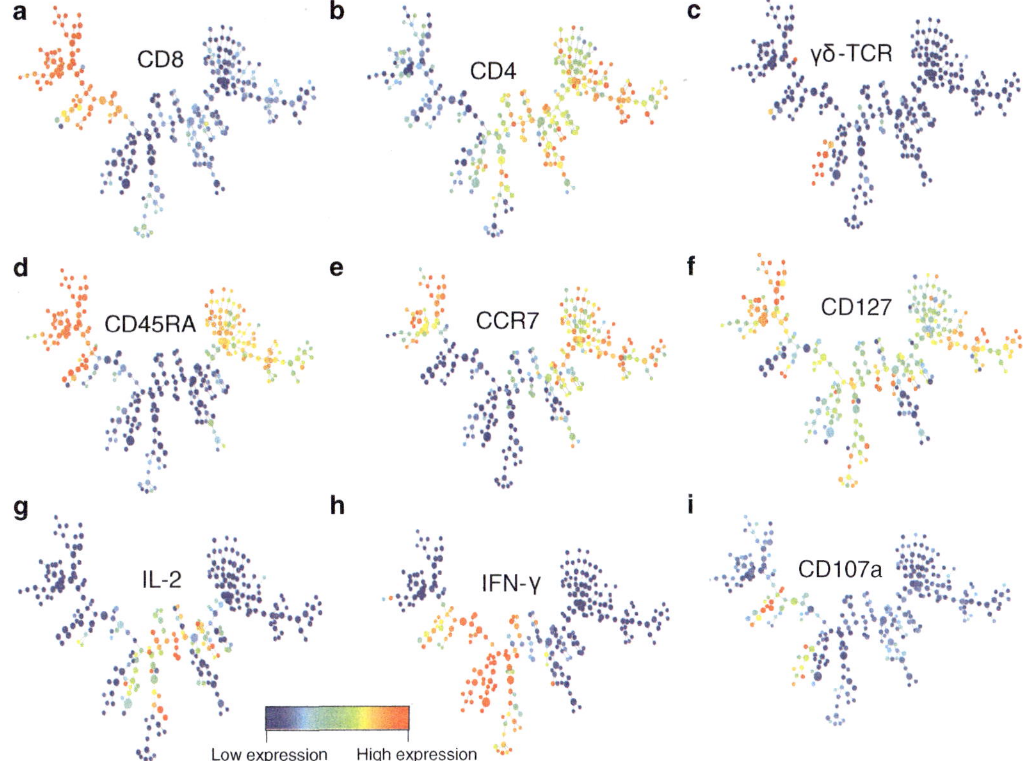


**Fig. 2** Example SPADE analysis of human peripheral blood T cells. Using a single PMA + ionomycin-stimulated sample, FlowJo software is used to gate on single live CD14-CD19-CD16-CD56-CD3+ T cells (*see* Fig. 1a–d). These events were exported as a new .fcs file and used for subsequent SPADE analysis. For this example only uninducible makers were used for tree hierarchical clustering and tree building [14, 15]. After clustering, default arrangement of nodes was used. For each plot the size of the node represents the relative number of cells in the cluster and the color of the node represents the relative median expression of each marker. (**a**–**d**) Examples of uninducible markers used for tree building shown ((**a**) CD8, (**b**) CD4, (**c**) γδTCR, (**d**) CD45RA, (**e**) CCR7, (**f**) CD127)). (**g**–**i**) The median intensities of example inducible markers not used for tree building also shown ((**g**) IL-2, (**h**) IFN-γ, (**i**) CD107a))

with this method). Based on this analysis the relationships between various populations of T cells can be inferred. Then, as illustrated in Fig. 2, the functional capacities of each of these populations can also be determined.

## 4 Notes

1. Use filter tips for addition of all reagents to prevent cross-contamination of heavy metal solutions; spin speed is at 14,000 × *g* for all protein concentration steps.
2. Anti-fluorophore secondary antibodies can be used to add flexibility to the mass cytometry panel. Anti-APC and anti-FITC antibodies can also be used for this purpose. This approach

can be particularly useful for antibodies that are not amenable to direct conjugation or to amplify signal of weakly staining antibodies.

3. These metal isotopes indicated by * are isotopes that need special consideration. Except for Dy-162 all of these isotopes are purchased from Trace Science, Inc. For all of these, including Dy-162 significant but minimal (less than ~1–5 %) contamination is detected in neighboring (+1 or −1 amu channels). Thus, the panel should be set up to accommodate this and interpretation of the data should take this into consideration. Similarly, oxidation can cause bleed-over of signal into the +16 amu channel for any of the isotopic labels, which can be a concern for high-abundance markers. For instance, some background Dy-162 can be detected in cells that are stained with Nd-146-labeled anti-CD8. This is ok for this panel because $CD8^+$ T cells can be analyzed separately from other T cells when evaluating IL-4 expression.
4. Like anti-fluorophore-labeled antibodies, heavy metal-conjugated streptavidin can be used to amply difficult-to-conjugate or weakly staining antibodies. *See* Newell et al. [5, 6] for more details about the preparation of this reagent. Alternatively, an anti-biotin antibody can be used as a secondary as sold by DVS Sciences, Inc.
5. Centrifugation spins should be done at 1,500 RPM (520 RCF) in a hanging bucket centrifuge adapted for use with 96-well plates for 2 min. Supernatant is removed by flicking forcefully into a bleach-containing bucket lined with paper towels (careful to avoid splashing). Afterwards, to remove additional supernatant, the plates are dabbed onto a dry paper towel.
6. Although the number of wash steps in this protocol may seem excessive, it is important to remove unbound metals that are free in solution in order to reduce background signal. Cells are washed in water to reduce the amount of salt introduced into the mass cytometer. As the cells are fixed twice during this protocol, this is not a problem. In addition, the cells pelleted in water are stable and can be run within a few weeks when stored at 4 °C.
7. Because of the duration of signal detected for each cell and the way that single cells are identified by mass cytometry, cell doublets are often detected. This can be minimized by several approaches. First, slow acquisition rates can help to reduce doublets by reducing the chance of two cells being coincidentally detected. Secondly, the number of double-cell events can be reduced by cells by gating on DNA content and "cell length." Double-cell events will have a higher DNA signal and can also have higher cell-length values. The use of mass tag

barcoding (not described here) [4] when not all possible barcodes are used can also greatly reduce the number double-cell events.

8. When comparing T cell phenotypes and function before and after stimulation, it is important to be aware of cell surface markers that change within the 3-h stimulation period. For instance, even though the cleavage is blocked in this protocol with TAPI-2, some reduction of CD62L will be observed. In addition, T cell receptor (CD3) and CD4 levels will also be reduced to varying degrees with PMA+ionomycin vs. CD3 +/− CD28 stimulation.

## Acknowledgments

We thank members of the Mark Davis, Garry Nolan, and Holden Maecker labs for their contributions of information about mass cytometry theory, usage, and experiences with various monoclonal antibodies leading to the development of this protocol. We also thank the mass cytometry platform users at the Singapore Immunology Network for assistance in validating this method, especially members of the Gennaro De Libero lab. Core funding through the Singapore Immunology Network supported this work.

### References

1. Bandura DR et al (2009) Mass cytometry technique for real time single cell multitarget immunoassay based on inductively coupled plasma time-of-flight mass spectrometry. Anal Chem 81(16):6813–6822
2. Bendall SC et al (2011) Single-cell mass cytometry of differential immune and drug responses across a human hematopoietic continuum. Science 332(6030):687–696
3. Krutzik PO, Nolan GP (2006) Fluorescent cell barcoding in flow cytometry allows high-throughput drug screening and signaling profiling. Nat Methods 3(5):361–368
4. Bodenmiller B et al (2012) Multiplexed mass cytometry profiling of cellular states perturbed by small-molecule regulators. Nat Biotechnol 30(9):858–867
5. Newell EW et al (2012) Cytometry by time-of-flight shows combinatorial cytokine expression and virus-specific cell niches within a continuum of CD8+ T cell phenotypes. Immunity 36(1):142–152
6. Newell EW et al (2013) Combinatorial tetramer staining and mass cytometry analysis facilitate T-cell epitope mapping and characterization. Nat Biotechnol 31(7):623–629
7. Newell EW, Lin W (2013) High-dimensional analysis of human CD8 T cell phenotype, function, and antigen specificity. Curr Top Microbiol Immunol 377:67–84
8. Jabbari A, Harty JT (2006) Simultaneous assessment of antigen-stimulated cytokine production and memory subset composition of memory CD8 T cells. J Immunol Methods 313(1–2):161–168
9. Betts MR et al (2003) Sensitive and viable identification of antigen-specific CD8+ T cells by a flow cytometric assay for degranulation. J Immunol Methods 281(1–2):65–78
10. Fienberg HG et al (2012) A platinum-based covalent viability reagent for single-cell mass cytometry. Cytometry A 81(6):467–475
11. Fuss IJ et al (2009) Isolation of whole mononuclear cells from peripheral blood and cord blood. In: Coligan JE et al (eds) Current protocols in immunology. Wiley, New York, NY, Chapter 7: p. Unit7 1
12. Yokoyama WM, Thompson ML, Ehrhardt RO (2012) Cryopreservation and thawing of cells. In: Coligan JE et al (eds) Current protocols in immunology. Wiley, New York, NY, Appendix 3: p. 3G

13. Leipold MD, Maecker HT (2012) Mass cytometry: protocol for daily tuning and running cell samples on a CyTOF mass cytometer. J Vis Exp 69:e4398
14. Linderman MD et al (2012) CytoSPADE: high-performance analysis and visualization of high-dimensional cytometry data. Bioinformatics 28(18):2400–2401
15. Qiu P et al (2011) Extracting a cellular hierarchy from high-dimensional cytometry data with SPADE. Nat Biotechnol 29(10): 886–891

# Chapter 8

# Detection of NF-κB Pathway Activation in T Helper Cells

**Oliver Gorka, Stefan Wanninger, and Jürgen Ruland**

## Abstract

Upon activation of CD4+ T helper cells the transcription factor complex NF-κB becomes activated and its subunits are able to translocate to the nucleus. There, the dimerized proteins regulate the transcription of for example cytokine and pro-survival genes. This process is of central importance for a proper function of T helper cells as its loss causes severe immunodeficiency, whereas its deregulation can contribute to lymphomagenesis or autoimmunity. In this protocol we describe four methods to investigate NF-κB activation in T helper cells by testing (1) the assembly of the Carma1-Malt1-Bcl10 complex by co-immunoprecipitation, (2) the activation of the IKK complex and the degradation of IκBα by western blot analysis, (3) the degradation of IκBα by intracellular flow cytometry, and (4) the nuclear translocation and DNA binding activity of NF-κB by nonradioactive electrophoretic mobility shift assay (EMSA).

**Key words** NF-κB, T Helper cells, Western blotting, Intracellular flow cytometry, EMSA, Co-immunoprecipitation, IκBα, IKK complex, CBM complex

## 1 Introduction

The activation of T helper cells is a complex and tightly regulated process that is crucial for proper adaptive immune responses. Full activation of a naïve T cell requires the specific binding of the T cell receptor to a cognate peptide-MHC class II complex and an additional co-stimulatory signal, which is also provided by the antigen-presenting cell through the CD28 co-receptor. Briefly, both events together induce a rapid cascade of intracellular signaling events including phosphorylation of immunoreceptor tyrosine-based activation motifs (ITAMs), activation of Src family kinases and scaffold proteins which activate for example phospholipase C (PLC) for cleaving phosphatidylinositol 4,5-bisphosphate ($PIP_2$) to inositol-1,4,5-triphosphate ($IP_3$) and diacylglycerol (DAG). $IP_3$ binding to $IP_3$-sensitive $Ca^{2+}$ channels induces release of stored $Ca^{2+}$ from the endoplasmic reticulum, whereas DAG promotes the activation of protein kinase C θ (PKCθ) at the inner membrane of the T cell [1]. Active PKCθ phosphorylates Carma1 (Card11) within its linker region and induces conformational changes that

Ari Waisman and Burkhard Becher (eds.), *T-Helper Cells: Methods and Protocols*, Methods in Molecular Biology, vol. 1193, DOI 10.1007/978-1-4939-1212-4_8, © Springer Science+Business Media New York 2014

enable Carma1 to interact with the preformed Bcl10/Malt1 complex [2, 3]. Upon the assembly of Carma1, Bcl10, and Malt1 into the so-called CBM complex, IKK proteins become phosphorylated and in turn mediate the phosphorylation of IκBα, which is subsequently ubiquitinated and degraded by the proteasome [4]. In the absence of stimulatory signals, NF-κB subunits are complexed with IκBα in the cytosol but are set free upon IκBα degradation and can translocate to the nucleus [5]. The NF-κB family comprises five related transcription factors, namely RelA (p65), p50, p52, RelB, and cRel. All NF-κB proteins contain a Rel-homology domain (RHD) that mediates protein-protein interactions for the formation of homodimers and/or heterodimers. Only RelA, RelB, and cRel contain transactivation domains (TAD) for activating the transcription of target genes. In contrast, p50 and p52 lack this ability and their homodimers are considered to repress target gene expression [5]. After translocation into the nucleus, NF-κB homodimers and/or heterodimers can bind to specific NF-κB DNA consensus sequences controlling transcription of cytokines or pro-survival factors such as Bcl-xl [6].

Here we describe four different methods to investigate some of the above-mentioned signaling events in detail. First, we focus on the formation of the CBM complex after T cell activation with PMA (Phorbol-12-myristate-13-acetate) and Ionomycin. Immunoprecipitation of Bcl10 and subsequent immunoblot analysis allows for monitoring the assembly of the CBM complex. Second, cell lysates of CD4+ T cells that are stimulated in a time-course experiment can be analyzed by western blotting for the phosphorylation of IKK proteins and IκBα and for the subsequent degradation of IκBα. Additionally, we describe a flow cytometry-based method to monitor IκBα degradation by intracellular stainings and FACS analysis. The cytoplasmic signaling events of an activated T cell via the CBM complex eventually lead to translocation of NF-κB subunits to the nucleus of a cell. Therefore, we finally describe a method to detect translocation of transcriptions factors to the nucleus, by isolation of nuclear fractions from T helper cells and their analysis by NF-κB-specific EMSA.

Taken together, the presented methods are of general interest in the field of T helper cell biology and provide scientist with helpful protocols to further investigate signaling events leading to the assembly of the CBM complex and the activation of NF-κB.

## 2 Materials

### 2.1 Required Materials for All Described Methods

1. Red blood cell (RBC) lysis buffer.
2. CD4 T cell isolation Kit II, mouse (Miltenyi Biotec).
3. Resting medium: RPMI 1640, 1 % FCS or 1 % BSA (w/v), 2 mM L-glutamine.

4. Reagents for T cell stimulation: 1 mM PMA (Phorbol-12-myristate-13-acetate) and 1 mM Ionomycin stock solutions in DMSO; Prepare 2× dilutions in resting medium to obtain a final concentration of 100 nM PMA and 250 nM Ionomycin during stimulation (*see* **Note 1**).

### 2.2 Co-immunoprecipitation (Co-IP) of the CBM Complex in T Cells

1. Co-IP Buffer: 50 mM HEPES (pH 7.5), 10 % glycerol (v/v), 0.1 % Triton X-100 (v/v), 1 mM DTT, 150 mM NaCl, 2 mM MgCl2 in deionized $H_2O$. Add fresh before use: 1× protease inhibitor cocktail.
2. Antibodies used for Co-IP: Anti-Bcl10 antibody (clone C-17, goat polyclonal IgG, Santa Cruz), Affinipure Goat Anti-Rat IgG isotype control (H+L, Jackson Immuno Research).
3. Protein G Sepharose 4 Fast Flow (GE Healthcare).
4. Antibodies used for western blotting: anti-Bcl10 (clone C78F1, CST), anti-Carma1 (clone 1D12, CST), anti-Malt1 as described in [7], anti-β-actin.
5. Western blotting materials as described in Subheading 2.3.

### 2.3 Western Blotting

1. PVDF Transfer membrane (Amersham Hybond-P, GE Healthcare).
2. Whatman paper.
3. CHAPS lysis buffer: 30 mM Tris–HCl (pH 7.5), 150 mM NaCl, 1 % CHAPS (w/v), in deionized $H_2O$. Add fresh before use: 1 μM PMSF, 1 μM DTT, 1× protease inhibitor cocktail.
4. 5× Laemmli buffer: 250 mM Tris–HCl (pH 6.8), 25 % glycerol, 10 % β-mercaptoethanol, 5 % SDS, 0.1 % bromophenol blue (w/v).
5. 10× TBS buffer: 200 mM Tris, 1.37 M NaCl in deionized $H_2O$, adjust pH to 7.4.
6. 1× TBST buffer: Dilute 10× TBS buffer in deionized $H_2O$ and add 0.1 % Tween-20.
7. Methanol.
8. 10× Running buffer: 250 mM Tris, 1.92 M glycine, 1 % SDS in deionized $H_2O$.
9. 10× Transfer buffer (for semi-dry blotting): 480 mM Tris, 390 mM glycine, 0.315 % SDS in deionized $H_2O$. When diluting 1× Transfer buffer freshly add 20 % methanol upon preparation.
10. Prestained protein ladder.
11. 10 % SDS-Polyacrylamide gel (Volumes for two minigels of 8.3 cm × 7.3 cm × 1 mm).

    Stacking gel: 3 mL deionized $H_2O$, 1.2 mL 0.5 M Tris–HCl (pH 6.6), 0.7 mL 30 % acrylamide/bisacrylamide solution, 25 μL 20 % SDS solution, add briefly before pouring the gel 25 μL 10 % APS solution and 5 μL TEMED (*N, N, N, N'* tetramethyl-ethylenediamine).

Running gel: 4.1 mL deionized $H_2O$, 2.5 mL 1.5 M Tris–HCl (pH 8.8), 3.3 mL 30 % acrylamide/bisacrylamide solution, 50 μL 20 % SDS solution, add briefly before pouring the gel 50 μL 10 % APS solution and 5 μL TEMED.

12. Protein electrophoresis equipment and semi-dry blotting apparatus (*see* **Note 2**).
13. Western blot blocking buffer: 5 % bovine serum albumin (w/v, Albumin Fraction V) in TBST.
14. Antibodies used for western blotting: rabbit anti-mouse pIKK alpha/beta (Ser176/180, clone 16A6, CST), rabbit anti-mouse p-IκBα (Ser32, clone 14D4, CST), rabbit anti-mouse IκBα (#9242, CST), rabbit anti-mouse β-actin (Sigma), anti-rabbit HRP (#7074, CST).
15. ECL solution.

### 2.4 Intracellular Flow Cytometry

1. FACS buffer: 3 % FCS in 1× PBS.
2. Paraformaldehyde (PFA), 4 %.
3. 75 % methanol in PBS.
4. Antibodies used for flow cytometry: anti-CD4 APC (clone GK1.5, eBioscience), anti-IκBα (clone L35A5, CST), anti-mouse $IgG_1$ FITC antibody (clone A85-1, eBioscience), mouse $IgG_1$ isotype control antibody (clone 3.6.2.8.1, eBioscience).
5. 96 U-well plates cell culture plates and 96 V-well plates.

### 2.5 NF-κB Electrophoretic Mobility Shift Assay

1. Additional reagents for T cell stimulation: Affinipure Rabbit Anti-Syrian Hamster IgG (H + L, Jackson Immuno Research), anti-mouse CD3e (Clone 145-2C11, eBioscience), anti-mouse CD28 (Clone 37.51, eBioscience).
2. Buffer A: 10 mM HEPES (pH 7.9), 10 mM KCl, 0.1 mM EDTA, 0.1 mM EGTA in deionized $H_2O$. Add fresh before use: 1 mM PMSF, 1 mM DTT, 1× protease inhibitor cocktail.
3. Buffer C: 20 mM HEPES (pH 7.9), 0.4 M NaCl, 1 mM EDTA, 1 mM EGTA in deionized $H_2O$. Add fresh before use: 1 mM PMSF, 1 mM DTT, 1× protease inhibitor cocktail.
4. 10 % Nonidet P-40 in deionized $H_2O$.
5. 1.5 mL tube orbital shaker.
6. IR Dye 700 NF-κB consensus oligonucleotides (LI-COR Biosciences).
7. 10× Binding Buffer: 100 mM Tris, 500 mM KCl, 10 mM DTT in deionized $H_2O$, adjust to pH 7.5.

8. Poly(dI-dC), 1 μg/μL in 10 mM Tris, 1 mM EDTA in deionized $H_2O$ (pH 7.5).
9. DTT/Tween solution: 25 mM DTT, 2.5 % Tween-20 in deionized $H_2O$.
10. 10× Orange Loading Dye (LI-COR Biosciences).
11. Large format protein electrophoresis equipment.
12. Running buffer: 0.5× TBE (Tris/Borate/EDTA) diluted from 10× TBE (Invitrogen) (*see* **Note 3**).
13. 5 % polyacrylamide gel: 5 % acrylamide/bisacrylamide, 50 % 1× TBE in deionized $H_2O$, add briefly before pouring the gel 1 % ammonium persulfate and 0.5 % TEMED (*see* **Note 4**).
14. Odyssey Infrared Imaging System (LI-COR Biosciences).

## 3 Methods

### 3.1 Procedures Common to All Methods Described in the Following

1. Prepare a single cell suspension of mouse spleens and/or lymph nodes. Place 100 μm strainer in 6-well plates with 5 mL of resting medium. Carefully dissect lymph nodes, remove all fat remains, and place tissue into the cell strainer. Thoroughly mash tissue through the strainer by using a 3 mL syringe plunger. Collect cell suspension in a 15 mL tube, centrifuge (350 × *g*, 5 min, 4 °C) and discard supernatant.
2. Lyse red blood cells for 5 min by resuspending the cell pellet in 1 mL of RBC lysis buffer and incubate at room temperature. Stop lysis reaction by adding 10 mL resting medium and centrifuge (350 × *g*, 5 min, 4 °C). Discard supernatant.
3. Purify untouched CD4+ T cells by CD4 T cell isolation Kit II (Miltenyi Biotec) following manufacturer's protocol.
4. Count isolated T cells and check purity by FACS analysis after staining for CD4 (*see* **Note 5**).
5. Rest cells for 1 h in resting medium at 37 °C in a concentration of $1 \times 10^7$ cells/mL.
6. Freshly prepare stimuli and all required reagents (such as Co-IP buffer or lysis buffer). Prepare an icebox and chill PBS, FACS buffer and lysis buffers. Thaw lysis buffer supplements and place them on ice.

### 3.2 Co-immunoprecipitation of the CBM Complex in T Cells

1. Use $1.5–2 \times 10^7$ freshly isolated CD4+ T helper cells for each co-immunoprecipitation.
2. Stimulate samples by adding one volume of prewarmed 2× stimulation predilution to obtain a final concentration 100 nM PMA and 250 nM Ionomycin. Add the same volume of resting medium to samples that are left unstimulated.

3. Keep cells at 37 °C for 30–60 min.
4. Harvest and wash cells with ice-cold PBS. Transfer cell suspension to a fresh 1.5 mL tube and centrifuge (350 × *g*, 5 min, 4 °C).
5. Aspirate the supernatant and resuspend the cell pellet in 900 μL of cold Co-IP Lysis Buffer.
6. Incubate for 20 min on a spinning wheel at 4 °C.
7. Prepare 40–60 μL of Protein G Sepharose beads per sample in a fresh tube. Add 900 μL Co-IP buffer to the beads, centrifuge (1,000 × *g*, 5 min, 4 °C) and carefully aspirate the supernatant. Repeat this washing step three times (*see* **Note 6**).
8. Centrifuge the Co-IP lysates at full speed (20,817 × *g*, 10 min, 4 °C).
9. Transfer the supernatant into a fresh 1.5 mL tube.
10. Transfer an aliquot (30–50 μL) of each lysate and into a fresh 1.5 mL tube as input control. Add one volume of 2× Laemmli buffer and boil input control samples at 95 °C for 10 min. Freeze input control samples at −20 °C and use later for western blotting.
11. Add 20–30 μL of Protein G Sepharose (half the amount of washed beads per sample) to each Co-IP sample for preclearing. Fill up the tube containing the remaining beads with Co-IP buffer and store at 4 °C until the next day.
12. Incubate Co-IP samples for 1 h at 4 °C on a spinning wheel for preclearing.
13. Spin down all samples (1,000 × *g*, 5 min, 4 °C) and transfer supernatants into fresh tubes.
14. Add anti-Bcl10 antibody (1 μg/per sample) or an isotype control to the respective samples.
15. Incubate over night at 4 °C on a spinning wheel (*see* **Note 7**).
16. Add 20–30 μL of Protein G Sepharose beads (set aside at 4 °C from the previous day) and incubate mixture for 1 h at 4 °C on a spinning wheel.
17. Spin down samples (1,000 × *g*, 5 min, 4 °C) and carefully discard supernatant (*see* **Note 8**).
18. Wash Protein G Sepharose beads three times with 900 μL of chilled Co-IP Lysis buffer.
19. After the last washing step add 20–30 μL of 2× Laemmli Buffer to the beads and boil samples for 5 min at 95 °C.
20. Spin down briefly and freeze samples at −20 °C.
21. Pour 10 % SDS-Polyacrylamide gels and continue with western blotting standard procedure as described in Subheading 3.3 (*see* **Note 9**). A typical Co-IP western blotting result can be seen in Fig. 1.

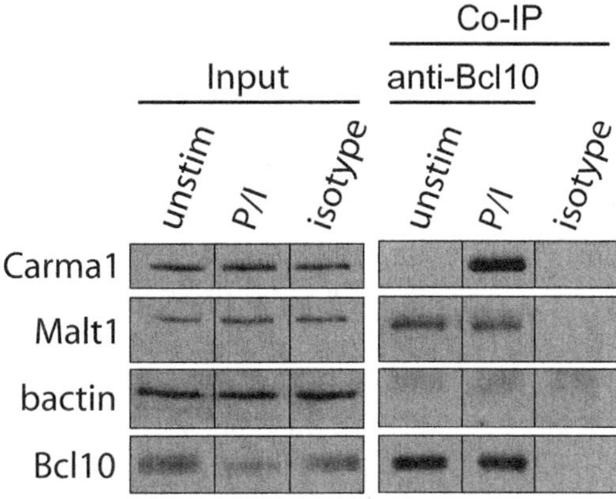


**Fig. 1** Co-Immunoprecipitation of the CBM complex in T cells. Anti-Bcl10 immunoprecipitation was carried out on freshly isolated CD4+ T cells either stimulated with PMA/Ionomycin for 30 min or left unstimulated. Western blots show input samples, anti-Bcl10 and isotype control immunoprecipitations using detection antibodies specific for Carma1, Malt1, β-actin and Bcl10. No interaction of Bcl10 with Carma1 can be detected in unstimulated CD4+ T cells. However, after stimulation with PMA/Ionomycin, Carma1 can be co-immunoprecipitated with Bcl10 and Malt1, indicating formation of the CBM complex

### *3.3 Analysis of NF-κB Activation in CD4+ T Helper Cells by Western Blotting*

1. Use at least $3 \times 10^6$ freshly isolated and rested CD4+ T cells per condition. We recommend including enough conditions for a time course experiment of 6 time points in a range between 0 and 60 min (e.g., 0, 2.5, 5, 10, 15, and 30 min).
2. Transfer 300 μL of CD4+ T cells at a concentration of $1 \times 10^7$ cells/mL to 1.5 mL tubes and place tube on a thermo-shaker set to 37 °C and 350 rpm.
3. Prewarm 2× stimulation predilution (100 nM PMA and 250 nM Ionomycin final concentration) at 37 °C.
4. Add 300 μL 2× stimulation predilution to every CD4+ T cell condition starting from the longest time point. Set an alarm clock after addition of all stimuli.
5. Stop stimulation reaction by adding 1 mL of ice-cold PBS to the respective tube and immediately placing the tube on ice.
6. After completion of the time course spin down samples in a precooled tabletop centrifuge (450 × *g*, 5 min, 4 °C) and carefully aspirate supernatants without disturbing the cell pellet.
7. Resuspend cell pellet in 30–50 μL of CHAPS lysis buffer plus supplements and keep lysates on ice for 30 min.
8. Spin down samples in a precooled tabletop centrifuge (20,817 × *g*, 15 min, 4 °C) and transfer lysates to fresh 1.5 mL tubes. Store lysates at −20 °C.

9. When continuing the experiment, gently thaw samples on ice and determine protein concentration of the samples by a method of choice (e.g., BCA or Bradford assay).
10. Pour 10 % SDS-polyacrylamide gels with 10 or 15 pocket gel combs depending of the number of samples.
11. Transfer 5–10 μg protein lysates per western blot to a fresh tubes and place on ice.
12. Add 5× Laemmli buffer to protein lysates and equilibrate volumes by addition of 1× Laemmli buffer to a maximal volume of 20 μL per western blot lane.
13. Boil lysates at 95 °C for 10 min on a preheated thermo-shaker at 450 rpm.
14. Briefly spin down tubes and place on ice.
15. Load gels with samples and protein ladder. Place protein ladder in first and last gel pockets.
16. Run gel with up to 100 V for stacking and up to 140 V for running gel phase.
17. For semi-dry blotting, prepare Whatman paper of appropriate size and wet all pre-cut papers in 1× Transfer buffer. Activate PVDF by methanol treatment (1 min), rinse briefly with deionized $H_2O$ and equilibrate membrane in 1× Transfer buffer.
18. After completion of the gel run, disassemble the running chambers and equilibrate the gel in 1× Transfer buffer for 2 min.
19. Stack moistened Whatman paper, PVDF membrane, and the gel in correct orientation inside of the blotting apparatus (*see* **Note 10**) and let it run at 25 V for 90 min.
20. After blotting the transfer can be tested by Ponceau S stain of the blot (*see* **Note 11**).
21. Block membrane with freshly prepared 5 % BSA (w/v) in TBST for 1 h at room temperature on a shaker.
22. If membranes are used with more than one primary antibody, cut them horizontally according to the respective size of you proteins of interest (*see* **Note 12**).
23. Incubate membranes in freshly diluted primary antibody solutions according to the manufacturer's recommendations in 5 % BSA in TBST at 4 °C over night either shaking or rolling.
24. Wash membranes three times for 5 min with a sufficient volume of TBST buffer.
25. Incubate membranes in a freshly diluted secondary antibody solution according to the manufacturer's recommendations in 5 % BSA in TBST at room temperature either shaking or rolling for 1 h.

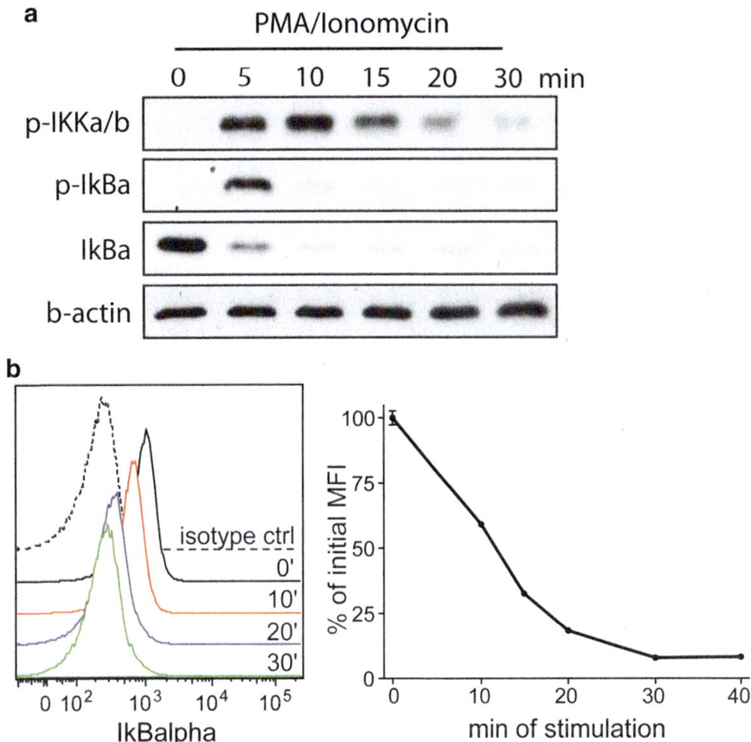


**Fig. 2** Analysis of NF-κB pathway activation by western blotting and intracellular flow cytometry. (**a**) Lysates of freshly isolated CD4+ T cells stimulated with PMA/Ionomycin in a time-course experiment show rapid phosphorylation of IKKα/β and IκBα. IκBα phosphorylation is immediately followed by its degradation. In (**b**) IκBα degradation is monitored by intracellular flow cytometry for total IκBα. The *left plot* shows stacked histogram overlays of IκBα signals at indicated time-points after PMA/Ionomycin stimulation, whereas the *right plot* shows the corresponding MFI values as percentage of the MFI measured in unstimulated T cells

26. Wash membranes five times for 5 min with sufficient TBST buffer and conclude the washing procedure by rinsing the membrane with 1× TBS.
27. Incubate membranes with ECL solution and expose to a photo film or detect emitted light by a CCD camera device. Figure 2a shows blotted lysates of PMA/Iono stimulated T cells from a time-course experiment.

#### 3.4 Intracellular Flow Cytometric Analysis of IκBα Degradation

1. Use $1 \times 10^6$ freshly isolated and rested CD4+ T cells per condition (*see* **Note 13**). We recommend including enough conditions for a time course experiment of at least 6 time points in a range between 0 and 60 min (e.g., 0′, 5′, 10′, 15′, 20′, and 30′).
2. Prepare a 96 U-well cell culture plate and transfer 100 μL of a $1 \times 10^7$ cells/mL suspension to each well used in the experiment and keep plate at 37 °C.

3. Prewarm 2× stimulation predilution (100 nM PMA and 250 nM Ionomycin final concentration) at 37 °C.
4. Add 100 μL 2× stimulation predilution to every CD4+ T cell stimulation condition starting from the longest time point. For unstimulated cells add 100 μL resting medium to the respective well. Set an alarm clock after addition of all stimuli and place 96-well plate to 37 °C.
5. Stop stimulation reaction by adding 100 μL of 4 % PFA to the respective well after each time point. Mix briefly by pipetting up and down. Place 96-well plate back to 37 °C.
6. After addition of PFA to the last time point incubate plate for another 15 min at 37 °C.
7. Prepare 75 % methanol in PBS and place on ice.
8. Transfer fixed cells to a 96 V bottom well plate and centrifuge (350×*g*, 5 min, 4 °C).
9. Discard supernatant, wash cells with 200 μL FACS buffer and centrifuge (350×*g*, 5 min, 4 °C). Repeat washing step.
10. An optional extracellular staining of the cells can be included now. Dilute a fluorophore-labeled anti-mouse CD4 antibody in FACS buffer according to the manufacturer's recommendation and incubate for 15 min at 4 °C (*see* **Note 14**).
11. After incubation centrifuge plate (350×*g*, 5 min, 4 °C), discard supernatant and wash cells twice with 200 μL FACS buffer.
12. Permeabilize cells by addition and of 200 μL ice-cold 75 % methanol. Resuspend and incubate cells for 20 min at 4 °C.
13. For intracellular staining dilute anti-IκBα (L35A5) and mouse $IgG_1$ isotype control antibodies in FACS buffer according to manufacturer's recommendation (*see* **Note 15**).
14. After permeabilization with methanol, centrifuge plate (350×*g*, 5 min, 4 °C), discard supernatant and wash cells twice with 200 μL FACS buffer to remove residual methanol.
15. Resuspend cells in antibody dilutions for intracellular staining and incubate for 30 min at 4 °C.
16. After incubation with primary intracellular antibodies, centrifuge plate (350×*g*, 5 min, 4 °C), discard supernatant, and wash cells twice with 200 μL FACS buffer.
17. Dilute the secondary anti-mouse $IgG_1$ FITC antibody according to the manufacturer's recommendation in FACS buffer (*see* **Note 16**).
18. Resuspend cells in secondary antibody dilution incubate for 30 min at 4 °C.
19. After incubation with the secondary intracellular antibody, centrifuge plate (350×*g*, 5 min, 4 °C), discard supernatant, and wash cells twice with 200 μL FACS buffer.

20. Resuspend cells in FACS buffer and transfer them to FACS tubes.
21. During flow cytometric analysis make sure to acquire at least 20,000 cells per condition (*see* **Note 17**).
22. For analysis, histogram overlays or calculated mean/median fluorescent intensity (MFI) values of the respective fluorochrome detector channel can be used (*see* **Note 18**). Compare Fig. 2b.

### 3.5 Detection of Nuclear NF-κB in CD4+ T Helper Cells by EMSA

1. For pre-coating of cell culture plates for plate-bound T cell stimulation incubate 6-well cell culture plates with 1 mL 10 μg/mL Affinipure Rabbit Anti-Syrian Hamster IgG in PBS for at least 1 h at 37 °C or over night at 4 °C. Aspirate buffer and wash with PBS. Dilute anti-mouse CD3e antibody in PBS to a final concentration of 5 μg/mL, add to wells and incubate for 1 h at 37 °C. Aspirate buffer and wash with PBS. Dilute 2× concentrated soluble anti-mouse CD28 (4 μg/mL) in resting medium and add to wells. The final anti-CD28 concentration will be 2 μg/mL.
2. Use $5 \times 10^6$–$1 \times 10^7$ freshly isolated and rested CD4+ T cells per condition.
3. Stimulate samples by adding one volume of prewarmed 2× stimulation predilution to obtain a final concentration 100 nM PMA and 250 nM Ionomycin. Add the same volume of resting medium to samples that are left unstimulated.

   In case of plate-bound anti-CD3 and soluble anti-CD28 antibody stimulation add one volume cells to pre-coated cell culture plates filled with one volume 2× concentrated soluble anti-CD28 antibody.
4. Spin down plates at 450 × *g* for 2 min and incubate at 37 °C for the course of stimulation (between 0.5 and 8 h).
5. Harvest cells and transfer to a fresh 1.5 mL tube (*see* **Note 19**).
6. Centrifuge tubes in a tabletop centrifuge (350 × *g*, 5 min, 4 °C).
7. Aspirate the supernatant and wash cells by resuspending in ice-cold PBS and subsequent centrifugation (350 × *g*, 5 min, 4 °C).
8. Aspirate the supernatant and lyse the cells by resuspending them in chilled 800 μL Buffer A plus supplements.
9. Incubate for 15 min on ice.
10. Add 50 μL of 10 % Nonidet P-40.
11. Let samples shake for 5 min with full speed on a 1.5 mL tube orbital shaker.
12. Centrifuge samples with full speed (20,817 × *g*, 10 min, 4 °C).
13. Take off supernatant (cytoplasmic fraction) by pipetting and collect in a new tube if needed for further analysis.

14. Wash nucleic pellet by carefully adding 200 μL of Buffer A. Do not resuspend.
15. Transfer the transparent nuclear pellet into a fresh precooled tube using a pipet tip.
16. Add 40 μL of Buffer C (increase volume according to cell number and pellet size).
17. Incubate samples at least 30 min on an orbital shaker with full speed.
18. Centrifuge samples with full speed (20,817 × *g*, 10 min, 4 °C).
19. Harvest supernatant (nuclear fraction) into a precooled 1.5 mL tube.
20. Freeze nuclear fraction samples in liquid nitrogen and store them at −80 °C.
21. When continuing the experiment, gently thaw samples on ice and determine protein concentration of the samples by a method of choice.
22. Use 5 μg of each nuclear extract to set up binding reaction (*see* **Note 20**). Mix nuclear extract with 2 μL 10× binding buffer, 1 μL poly(dI-dC), 2 μL DTT/Tween solution, 1 μL 1 % NP-40, 1 μL IRDye 700 NF-κB probe and fill up with deionized water to a total volume of 20 μL.
23. Incubate for 20–30 min in the dark at room temperature.
24. In the meantime pour a large 5 % polyacrylamide gel for EMSA applications.
25. Place gel into a running chamber using 0.5× TBE as running buffer.
26. Wash and clean pockets thoroughly by flushing with running buffer using a syringe.
27. Add 2 μL 10× Orange Loading Dye to the samples and mix briefly.
28. Load samples into pockets (*see* **Note 21**).
29. Run gel at 150–200 V for approximately 2 h. Do not let the unbound probe run out of the gel. Since the IRDye is sensitive to light, protect the whole chamber from light by covering it (*see* **Note 22**).
30. Scan the gel in an Odyssey Imager without removing the glass plates. Clean glass plates thoroughly before scanning. Adjust the Odyssey settings (especially the focus offset) according to manufacturer's recommendation. A typical result can be seen in Fig. 3.

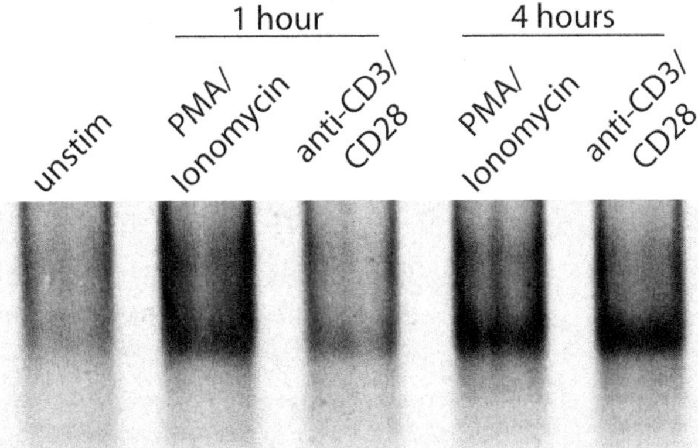


**Fig. 3** Detection of nuclear NF-κB in CD4+ T helper cells by EMSA. Freshly isolated CD4+ T cells were stimulated with PMA/Ionomycin or plate-bound anti-CD3 plus soluble anti-CD28 for 1 and 4 h or were left unstimulated. Stimulation with anti-CD3/CD28 or PMA/Ionomycin leads to translocation of NF-κB subunits to the nucleus and binding of NF-κB transcription factors to IR Dye 700 NF-κB consensus oligonucleotides. The signal strength increases with stimulation time and PMA/Ionomycin induces faster and stronger NF-κB nuclear translocation than stimulation with anti-CD3/CD28

## 4 Notes

1. The PMA/Ionomycin working concentration ranges for 10 nM to 1 μM. For this protocol we use a relatively high concentration resulting in rapid and full activation of the studied pathways. For more physiological stimulation of T cells, plate-bound anti-CD3 and anti-CD28 antibodies can be used as described in Subheading 3.5.
2. In this protocol we use semi-dry blotting for all western blot applications. This blotting procedure is known to produce reliable results for smaller proteins and is less time and buffer consuming than wet blot applications. Nevertheless, both semi-dry and wet blotting work fine for the detection of the proteins described in this protocol.
3. 10× TBE solution tends to precipitate at room temperature after a period of time. If precipitates become visible we recommend autoclaving of the whole solution including the precipitated particles.
4. For EMSA application long gels are usually used to completely separate free oligonucleotide probes and shifted bands. The gel apparatus used for the experiments shown in

this protocol was 18 cm × 16 cm in size with 1.5 mm spacing and 15 pocket combs.

5. This step is crucial to verify the presence of a purified CD4+ T cell population for all subsequent experiments in this protocol. Only continue with experiments if purity of CD4+ T cells is about 95 % or greater.
6. Repeat this washing step three times to completely remove the ethanol from the storage solution. Make sure not to disturb the beads during aspiration.
7. If unwanted background signal or unspecific binding is observed with overnight incubation it may be helpful to shorten incubation time.
8. Use a thin injection needle to remove all supernatant without loosing any Sepharose beads for all following steps.
9. Avoid the transfer of beads to the SDS-polyacrylamide gel when loading IP samples.
10. Thoroughly push out any trapped air from Whatman paper stacks by firmly rolling a 5 mL plastic pipette over it.
11. If incorrect blotting due to air bubbles or any kind of disturbance is visible, consider repeating the western blot.
12. For the proteins discussed in this protocol two membranes were prepared and cut. One membrane was cut at the height of 60 kDa and was used for p-IKKα/β (85–87 kDa) and p-IκBα (40 kDa) detection. The other membrane was cut at a height of 42 kDa and was taken for the detection of β-actin (45 kDa) and total IκBα (39 kDa). Antibody-dilutions can be stored and reused if 0.01–0.05 % sodium azide is added as a preservative.
13. This experimental procedure also works on total splenocytes or any other kind of cell mixture. In this case further populations must be distinguished by additional extracellular antibody stainings.
14. Some surface antigens are rapidly internalized upon stimulation. This effect can be overcome by permeabilization of the cells prior to staining procedure or antibody staining of the cells before stimulation.
15. Make sure to adjust the concentration of experimental and isotype control antibodies. Some companies do not provide the concentrations in their technical datasheets. Include the lot number of the respective antibody when requesting the concentration as concentrations may differ from a lot to another.
16. The anti-IκBα (L35A5) antibody has already become available as directly labeled antibody. By using a directly labeled antibody you can circumvent the need of secondary and isotype control antibodies.

17. Acquisition at low flow rates usually gives higher resolution during flow cytometric measurement.
18. Consider using median fluorescent intensity values if the population of interest does not show normal distribution.
19. T cells become adherent during plate-bound stimulation. Rinse and resuspend cells from cell culture plates with ice-cold PBS.
20. Antibodies against different NF-κB subunits can be included in the reaction to perform supershifts. This method is useful to determine specific binding of certain NF-κB subunits to oligonucleotide probes.
21. Loading the gel asymmetrically helps in terms of gel orientation.
22. EMSA running buffer (0.5× TBE) can be reused several times and can be stored at room temperature.

## Acknowledgments

The authors would like to thank Dr. Andreas Gewies for critical reading of the manuscript and all members of the laboratory for input and discussion.

### References

1. Smith-Garvin JE, Koretzky GA, Jordan MS (2009) T cell activation. Annu Rev Immunol 27:591–619. doi:10.1146/annurev.immunol.021908.132706
2. Matsumoto R, Wang D, Blonska M, Li H, Kobayashi M, Pappu B, Chen Y, Wang D, Lin X (2005) Phosphorylation of CARMA1 plays a critical role in T Cell receptor-mediated NF-kappaB activation. Immunity 23(6):575–585. doi:10.1016/j.immuni.2005.10.007
3. Sommer K, Guo B, Pomerantz JL, Bandaranayake AD, Moreno-Garcia ME, Ovechkina YL, Rawlings DJ (2005) Phosphorylation of the CARMA1 linker controls NF-kappaB activation. Immunity 23(6):561–574. doi:10.1016/j.immuni.2005.09.014
4. Ruland J, Duncan GS, Wakeham A, Mak TW (2003) Differential requirement for Malt1 in T and B cell antigen receptor signaling. Immunity 19(5):749–758
5. Hayden MS, Ghosh S (2004) Signaling to NF-kappaB. Genes Dev 18(18):2195–2224. doi:10.1101/gad.1228704
6. Ferch U, zum Buschenfelde CM, Gewies A, Wegener E, Rauser S, Peschel C, Krappmann D, Ruland J (2007) MALT1 directs B cell receptor-induced canonical nuclear factor-kappaB signaling selectively to the c-Rel subunit. Nat Immunol 8(9):984–991. doi:10.1038/ni1493
7. Ruefli-Brasse AA, French DM, Dixit VM (2003) Regulation of NF-kappaB-dependent lymphocyte activation and development by paracaspase. Science 302(5650):1581–1584. doi:10.1126/science.1090769

# Chapter 9

# Assessing the Suppressive Activity of Foxp3⁺ Regulatory T Cells

**Christian Thomas Mayer and Tim Sparwasser**

## Abstract

Foxp3⁺ regulatory T cells (Tregs) balance the mammalian immune system by mechanisms that are yet to be elucidated in their entirety. Methods employed to quantify the regulatory activity of Tregs in vitro are an important tool in cellular immunology, but can be technically demanding and subjected to variation. In this manuscript, we describe in detail a robust Treg suppression assay based on the flow cytometric quantification of both CD4⁺ and CD8⁺ effector T cell functions. This method can provide valuable insights into the immunosuppressive activity of Foxp3⁺ Tregs and is versatile with regard to genetic or pharmacologic manipulations. Additionally, novel regulatory immune cells can be characterized by using this assay.

**Key words** Foxp3, Treg, Suppression assay, Tolerance, Autoimmunity, Cancer

## 1 Introduction

A dysregulated immune system is potentially dangerous and must be controlled by immunological tolerance in order to prevent excessive inflammation and tissue destruction. Foxp3⁺ regulatory T cells (Tregs) have emerged as an essential layer of tolerance, e.g., by suppressing the activity of autoreactive lymphocytes and by modulating immune responses against pathogens through mechanisms that are still incompletely resolved [1, 2]. However, there is also evidence that Foxp3⁺ Tregs are instrumentalized by tumor cells and certain pathogens in order to evade protective immunity [2, 3]. Thus, a tight regulation of both the Treg compartment size and its immunosuppressive activity is essential for immune homeostasis. The underlying mechanisms are of great interest for the potential therapeutic manipulation of tolerance in humans.

In vitro methods for assessing the function of Tregs have been described shortly after the discovery of CD25 as a marker for CD4⁺ Tregs. These so-called suppression assays are based on the inhibition of T cell proliferation and/or cytokine production by co-culturing Tregs with responder T cells (Tresp) and antigen-presenting cells

Ari Waisman and Burkhard Becher (eds.), *T-Helper Cells: Methods and Protocols*, Methods in Molecular Biology, vol. 1193, DOI 10.1007/978-1-4939-1212-4_9, © Springer Science+Business Media New York 2014

(APCs). Robust suppression requires T cell receptor ligation on Tregs and is dependent on their physical contact with Tresp and/or APCs, whereas suppression can be abrogated by agonistic anti-CD28 co-stimulation [4, 5]. Consequently, Treg suppression assays have many variables that can influence the experimental results. These include the methods used for T cell and Treg isolation, the type and concentration of stimulatory agents, the type and number of APCs (which may vary in their co-stimulatory capacity), and the methods applied for the quantification of responder T cell function. In contrast to classical protocols based on $^{3}$H-thymidine incorporation for the detection of proliferation, multicolor flow cytometry allows for the simultaneous measurement of multiple parameters at a single-cell level.

Here we describe a flow cytometry-based Treg suppression assay using bone marrow-derived dendritic cells (GMCSF-DCs) as APCs, bacterial artificial chromosome (BAC)-transgenic DEREG mice for Foxp3$^{+}$ Treg isolation [6–8], and congenic mice for responder T cell isolation. This protocol includes the generation of GMCSF-DCs, isolation of T cells, setup of the suppression assay, and flow cytometric analysis. In contrast to assays with splenic APCs, this assay is more stable in our hands and has been successfully used to assess the suppressive function of Foxp3$^{+}$ Tregs and to characterize potential novel regulatory immune cells [9, 10].

## 2 Materials

All materials used for cell isolation and cell culture have to be sterile and should be handled in a sterile laminar flow hood. All reagents and buffers are stored at 4 °C if not stated otherwise.

### 2.1 Mice

6–8-week-old sex-matched DEREG mice, congenic CD45.1$^{+}$ wild-type (WT) mice, and CD45.2$^{+}$ WT mice (all on a C57Bl/6 background and housed under specific pathogen-free conditions; *see* **Notes 1** and **2**).

### 2.2 Cell Isolation and Cell Culture

1. Sterile Dulbecco's phosphate-buffered saline (DPBS).
2. Sterile DPBS containing 1 % heat-inactivated fetal calf serum (FCS; *see* **Note 3**) (isolation buffer).
3. Sterile DPBS containing 1 % heat-inactivated fetal calf serum and 2 mM EDTA (sorting buffer).
4. Red blood cell (RBC) lysis buffer: 150 mM ammonium chloride, 10 mM potassium hydrogen carbonate, 0.1 mM EDTA. Dissolve all reagents in 750 mL deionized water and adjust to pH 7.2–7.4. Add deionized water to 1 L and sterilize the buffer (0.22 μm filter).
5. 15 and 50 mL Falcon tubes.

6. 70 μm cell strainers.
7. Syringes and 27 G needles.
8. 70 % ethanol.
9. Dynabeads Untouched Mouse CD4 cells Kit (Invitrogen).
10. Dynabeads Untouched Mouse CD8 cells Kit (Invitrogen).
11. Dynamag-15 magnet (Invitrogen).
12. Anti-CD25-PE (clone PC61, eBioscience).
13. Anti-PE Microbeads (Miltenyi).
14. LS columns (Miltenyi).
15. MidiMACS separator and MACS MultiStand (Miltenyi).
16. Complete culture medium: RPMI 1640 supplemented with 10 % heat-inactivated fetal calf serum (FCS, *see* **Note 3**), 100 U/mL penicillin, 100 μg/mL streptomycin, and 50 μM β-mercaptoethanol.
17. 5(6)-Carboxyfluorescein diacetate *N*-succinimidyl ester (CFSE; *see* **Note 4**).
18. U-bottom 96-well cell culture plates.
19. Sterile 10 cm petri dishes.
20. Supernatant containing recombinant murine GMCSF [11] (*see* **Note 5**).
21. Anti-CD3ε (clone 145-2C11, functional grade).
22. Phorbol 12-myristate 13-acetate (PMA) and ionomycin. Store stock solutions at −20 °C.
23. 1,000× brefeldin A solution (eBioscience).

### 2.3 Flow Cytometry

1. V-bottom 96-well plates.
2. DPBS containing 1 % BSA and 2 mM EDTA (FACS buffer).
3. DPBS containing 1 % BSA, 2 mM EDTA, and 0.5 % saponin (permeabilization buffer).
4. Anti-CD16/CD32 supernatant (Fc block, clone 2.4G2, *see* **Note 6**).
5. Anti-CD4-Alexa647 (clone GK1.5, eBioscience, 1:200), anti-CD8α-eFluor450 (clone 53-6.7, eBioscience, 1:100), CD45.1-PE (clone A20, eBioscience, 1:400), IFN-γ-Alexa647 (clone XMG1.2, eBioscience, 1:100) (*see* **Note 7**).
6. 1 mg/mL propidium iodide (PI).
7. 2 mg/mL ethidium bromide monoazide (EMA) in dimethyl formamide. Store aliquots at −20 °C.
8. 4 % Paraformaldehyde (PFA) in PBS.
9. Polypropylene FACS tubes, 1.2 mL.

## 3 Methods

Centrifugation in Falcon tubes is routinely performed at 359 × *g* for 7 min at 4 °C. Centrifugation of V-bottom 96-well plates is done at 359 × *g* for 3 min at 4 °C. During cell isolation, work fast and keep buffers and cells on ice if not stated otherwise. Cultures are incubated at 37 °C, 5 % $CO_2$.

### 3.1 Generation of GMCSF-DCs

1. Isolate femurs and tibiae from a sacrificed $CD45.2^+$ WT mouse. Remove the remaining muscle tissue by careful rubbing with a tissue paper.
2. Sterilize intact bones for 1 min using 70 % ethanol in a petri dish. Wash the bones in sterile cold DPBS.
3. Place a 70 μm cell strainer into a 50 mL Falcon tube.
4. Grasp one bone with forceps and cut open both the ends with sterile scissors.
5. Penetrate one side of the bone with a syringe (best 27 G needle) and rinse the bone marrow with sterile cold DPBS into the cell strainer. Repeat this step from the other side of the bone until all the bone marrow is isolated and the bone appears whitish. Perform the **steps 4** and **5** with the remaining three bones.
6. Use the plunger of a 2 mL syringe to prepare a single-cell suspension and rinse the cell strainer with sterile cold DPBS.
7. Pellet the cells by centrifugation and discard the supernatant.
8. Resuspend cells in 1 mL of RBC lysis buffer and incubate for 1 min at room temperature. Add 9 mL of cold DPBS.
9. Take an aliquot for cell counting and pellet the cells. During centrifugation, determine the absolute cell number using a Neubauer counting chamber. Discard the supernatant after centrifugation.
10. Resuspend the cells in complete culture medium (pre-warmed to 37 °C). Decide on the number of plates to be cultured (one plate is sufficient for the described experiment; *see* **Note 8**).
11. Seed $2–4 \times 10^6$ cells in a sterile 10 cm petri dish. Add medium containing GMCSF supernatant (*see* **Note 5**) to a final volume of 10 mL. Culture at 37 °C.
12. On day 2, add 10 mL of complete culture medium pre-warmed to 37 °C.
13. On day 4, transfer 10 mL of the culture (without resuspending the cells) into a 50 mL Falcon tube and centrifuge.
14. Discard the supernatant and add 10 mL of fresh pre-warmed complete culture medium with GMCSF. Transfer back into the original petri dish and continue to culture at 37 °C.
15. Repeat **steps 13** and **14** on day 6.

16. Harvest the non-adherent cells on day 8 without exaggerated pipetting (*see* **Note 8**) and transfer the culture into a 50 mL Falcon tube. Centrifuge the cells and discard the supernatant.
17. Add 10 mL complete culture medium to wash the GMCSF-DCs. Centrifuge the cells and discard the supernatant. Repeat this washing step once and determine the cell number (*see* **Note 9**).
18. Resuspend at $6 \times 10^4$ cells/mL in complete culture medium.

### 3.2 Isolation of T Cells

1. Obtain spleen, peripheral lymph nodes, and mesenteric lymph nodes of a sacrificed CD45.1$^+$ WT mouse and pool the organs in a 70 μm cell strainer inserted into a 50 mL Falcon tube.
2. Use the plunger of a 2 mL syringe to prepare a single-cell suspension and rinse the cell strainer with isolation buffer.
3. Pellet the cells by centrifugation and discard the supernatant.
4. Resuspend the cells in 1 mL of RBC lysis buffer and incubate for 1 min at room temperature. Add 9 mL of isolation buffer.
5. Take an aliquot for cell counting and pellet the cells. During centrifugation, determine the absolute cell number using a Neubauer counting chamber. Discard the supernatant after centrifugation.
6. Follow the manufacturer's instructions for the untouched isolation of CD4$^+$ and CD8$^+$ T cells (*see* **Note 10**). One half of the cells are used for isolating CD4$^+$ T cells, and the other half to purify CD8$^+$ T cells.
7. Store the negatively selected CD8$^+$ T cells on ice.
8. Centrifuge the negatively selected CD4$^+$ T cells, discard the supernatant, and resuspend the cells in 1 mL isolation buffer.
9. Add 2.5 μL anti-CD25-PE and incubate for 10 min at 4 °C in the dark.
10. Add 9 mL isolation buffer, centrifuge the cells, and discard the supernatant.
11. Follow the manual of the anti-PE Microbeads (Miltenyi) and select CD25$^-$ cells by MACS.
12. Centrifuge CD4$^+$CD25$^-$ and CD8$^+$ T cells and resuspend them in 10 mL DPBS (without FCS).
13. Centrifuge again and resuspend the cells in 1 mL DPBS (without FCS).
14. Add 5 μM CFSE, mix rapidly, and incubate for 7 min at 37 °C in a water bath protected from light.
15. Add 9 mL complete culture medium, store for 5 min on ice, then centrifuge the cells, and discard the supernatant.
16. Wash twice with 10 mL complete culture medium.
17. Determine the cell number and resuspend CFSE$^+$ T cells at $1 \times 10^6$/mL in complete medium.

**Table 1**

**Pipetting scheme for the suppression assay**

| | CFSE+ T cells (1 × 10$^6$/mL) | GMCSF-DCs (6 × 10$^4$/mL) | Tregs (1 × 10$^6$/mL) | Anti-CD3ε (4 μg/mL) | Medium |
|---|---|---|---|---|---|
| Negative control | 50 μL | 50 μL | – | – | 100 μL |
| Positive control | 50 μL | 50 μL | – | 50 μL | 50 μL |
| Treg:T (1:1) | 50 μL | 50 μL | 50 μL | 50 μL | – |
| Treg:T (1:5) | 50 μL | 50 μL | 10 μL | 50 μL | 40 μL |

### 3.3 Isolation of Tregs

1. Follow **steps 1–5** of Subheading 3.2 (isolation of T cells) using two sacrificed DEREG mice (*see* **Notes 11** and **12**).
2. Resuspend the cells in 1 mL sterile sorting buffer.
3. Add Fc block (*see* **Note 6**) and incubate for 20 min at 4 °C.
4. Centrifuge, discard the supernatant, and resuspend the cells in 1 mL sorting buffer.
5. Add anti-CD4-Alexa647, mix, and incubate for 30 min at 4 °C in the dark.
6. Add 9 mL sorting buffer, centrifuge cells, and discard the supernatant.
7. Repeat **step 6**.
8. Resuspend cells in an appropriate volume of sorting buffer for FACS sorting.
9. Sort CD4$^+$eGFP$^+$ Tregs into a chilled 15 mL Falcon tube containing 1 mL pure FCS.
10. Determine the cell number and centrifuge.
11. Resuspend at $1 \times 10^6$ cells/mL in complete medium.

### 3.4 Suppression Assay

1. Prepare a stock solution of anti-CD3ε (4 μg/mL) in complete medium.
2. Prepare two 96-well U-bottom cell culture plates, one for CD4$^+$CD25$^-$ responder T cells and the other for CD8$^+$ responder T cells.
3. Set up the suppression assay (*see* Table 1). Negative controls contain responder T cells and DCs but no anti-CD3ε. Positive control wells receive responder T cells, DCs, and anti-CD3ε. The experimental samples contain responder T cells, DCs, anti-CD3ε, and Tregs at varying ratios of Tregs:responder T cells (*see* **Note 13**). The responder T cell number is kept constant and the final volume of each well is 200 μL. Set up each condition in triplicates. Prepare one additional negative

control and four additional positive control wells for adjusting the flow cytometer settings.

4. Incubate the plate at 37 °C for 5 days (*see* **Note 14**).

### 3.5 Staining of CD8$^+$ T Cells

1. Add 100 ng/mL PMA and 1 µg/mL ionomycin to all wells and mix. Incubate for 3 h at 37 °C.
2. Add 1× brefeldin A to all wells and mix. Incubate for an additional 3 h at 37 °C.
3. Transfer the cells into a V-bottom 96-well plate and centrifuge.
4. Discard the supernatant.
5. Add 200 µL FACS buffer, centrifuge the plate, and discard the supernatant to wash the cells.
6. Resuspend the cells in 50 µL FACS buffer containing Fc block (*see* **Note 6**) and EMA (1:1,000 dilution).
7. Place the plate approximately 30 cm below a standard light source and expose for 20 min on ice.
8. Repeat **step 5** twice.
9. Resuspend the cells in 50 µL FACS buffer containing anti-CD8α-eFluor450 and anti-CD45.1-PE. Add 50 µL FACS buffer to one additional negative control and to one additional positive control. Add 50 µL FACS buffer containing only anti-CD8α-eFluor450 or only anti-CD45.1-PE to one additional positive control. Incubate for 30 min at 4 °C in the dark.
10. Repeat **step 5** twice.
11. Resuspend the cells in 100 µL 2 % PFA in DPBS (without BSA and EDTA) and incubate for 20 min on ice in the dark.
12. Centrifuge the cells and discard the supernatant.
13. Wash the cells twice with 200 µL permeabilization buffer.
14. Add 50 µL permeabilization buffer containing anti-IFN-γ-Alexa647.
15. Incubate for 30 min at 4 °C in the dark.
16. Wash the cells twice with 200 µL permeabilization buffer.
17. Resuspend the cells in 100 µL FACS buffer and transfer into FACS tubes.
18. Proceed to flow cytometry.

### 3.6 Staining of CD4$^+$ T Cells

1. Transfer the cells into a V-bottom 96-well plate and centrifuge.
2. Discard the supernatant.
3. Add 200 µL FACS buffer, centrifuge the plate, and discard the supernatant to wash the cells.

4. Resuspend the cells in 50 μL FACS buffer containing Fc block (*see* **Note 6**).
5. Incubate the plate for 20 min at 4 °C.
6. Centrifuge the cells and discard the supernatant.
7. Resuspend the cells in 50 μL FACS buffer containing anti-CD4-Alexa647 and anti-CD45.1-PE (*see* **Note 15**). Add 50 μL FACS buffer to one additional negative control and to one additional positive control. Add 50 μL FACS buffer containing only anti-CD4-Alexa647 or only anti-CD45.1-PE to one additional positive control, respectively. Incubate for 30 min at 4 °C in the dark.
8. Repeat **step 3** twice.
9. Resuspend the cells in 100 μL FACS buffer containing PI (1:1,000) and transfer into FACS tubes.
10. Proceed to flow cytometry.

### 3.7 Flow Cytometry

1. Use the unstained positive and negative controls to adjust the voltages of all channels. Use the single stains to perform compensations where necessary (*see* **Note 16**).
2. Acquire the samples and save the data.
3. Analyze the fcs files with appropriate software. Gate on lymphocytes (FSC-A vs. SSC-A), single cells (SSC-W vs. SSC-A), and live cells (PE vs. PI/EMA; *see* **Note 17**). Then gate on $CD4^+CD45.1^+$ (*see* Fig. 1) or $CD8\alpha^+CD45.1^+$ responder T cells (*see* **Note 18**) and display histograms showing the CFSE dilution profile (*see* Figs. 1 and 2). For the restimulated $CD8^+CD45.1^+$ T cells, additionally display CFSE dilution vs. IFN-γ production (*see* Fig. 2). $Foxp3^+$ Tregs clearly suppress the proliferation of $CD4^+$ responder T cells (*see* Fig. 1). Interestingly, $Foxp3^+$ Tregs almost completely prevent IFN-γ production by $CD8^+$ Tresp cells, although the impact on proliferation is less pronounced when compared to the effects on $CD4^+$ Tresp proliferation (*see* Fig. 2).

## 4 Notes

1. For the described experiment, two DEREG mice, one $CD45.1^+$ WT mouse and one $CD45.2^+$ WT mouse, yield sufficient cell numbers. If additional conditions are included, the number of mice has to be increased accordingly. Other congenic strains such as Thy1.1 may be used instead of CD45.1. The use of congenic markers is strongly recommended for this assay because the CFSE signals of proliferated responder T cells and accessory cells might otherwise overlap (GMCSF-DCs induce stronger proliferation than splenic APCs). The assay can also

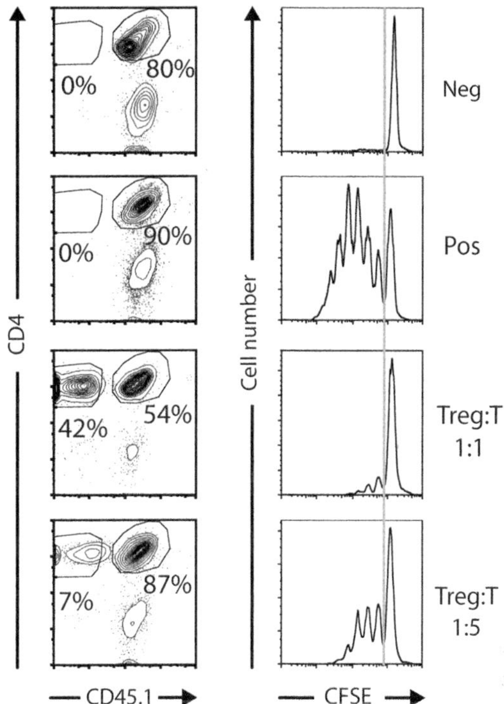


**Fig. 1** $CD4^+$ T cell suppression assay. The Treg suppression assay was analyzed by flow cytometry after 5 days of culture and live single cells were gated. Dot plots on the *left side* illustrate the gating on $CD4^+CD45.1^+$ responder T cells, whereas $CD4^+CD45.1^-$ cells represent Tregs added at varying ratios. The *right panels* show the CFSE dilution profiles of $CD4^+CD45.1^+$ responder T cells. Responder T cells without anti-CD3ε stimulation (Neg) or with stimulation but without added Tregs (Pos) served as controls. Reproduced from [9] with permission from Wiley

be easily performed on a Balb/c background (DEREG/Balb/c mice are available).

2. Here we only describe the classical suppression assay using polyclonal stimulation. However, the protocol may be easily adapted to perform alloreactive or antigen-specific suppression assays. Under these conditions, the T cell receptor ligation of responder T cells and Tregs can be separated.
3. We recommend to test and compare FCS batches from several providers (GMCSF-DC differentiation, DC activation, T cell proliferation) before ordering a particular batch.
4. Alternative proliferation dyes may be used. However, the antibody staining panel needs to be adjusted accordingly.
5. The concentration of GMCSF in the produced supernatant (complete RPMI 1640 medium) is batch dependant and requires previous testing for optimal GMCSF-DC generation. ELISA measurement (Mouse GMCSF Quantikine ELISA Kit, R&D)

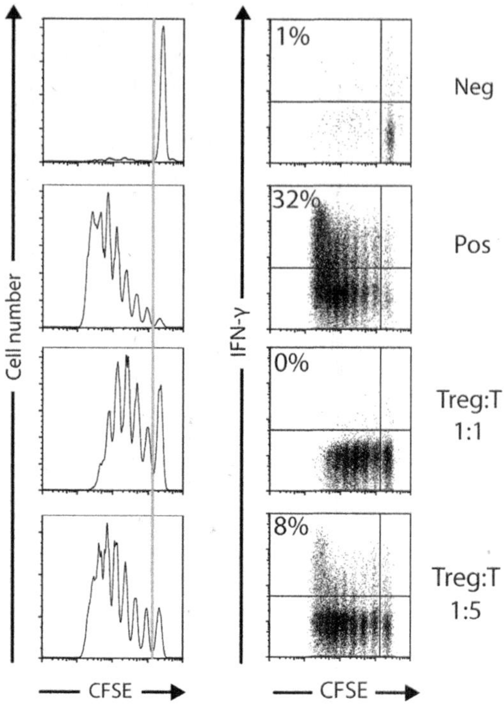


**Fig. 2** $CD8^+$ T cell suppression assay. The 5-day Treg suppression assay was restimulated for 6 h and analyzed by flow cytometry. Live $CD8^+CD45.1^+$ responder T cells were gated. The *left panels* show the CFSE dilution profiles. Dot plots on the *right side* display CFSE dilution vs. IFN-γ production of $CD8^+CD45.1^+$ responder T cells. Responder T cells without anti-CD3ε stimulation (Neg) or with stimulation but without added Tregs (Pos) served as controls. Reproduced from [9] with permission from Wiley

revealed that the final GMCSF concentration in our cultures approximates 6 ng/mL. The supernatant should not exceed 10 % of the total culture. Recombinant murine GMCSF (Peprotech) may be used alternatively at 20 ng/mL [12].

6. The concentration of Fc block in the produced supernatant is batch dependant and requires previous testing for successful application. Commercial anti-CD16/CD32 may be used as an alternative.
7. The antibody dilutions may vary depending on the flow cytometer used. Antibodies with different fluorochromes or from different suppliers should be titrated before performing the assay.
8. Non-adherent cells may be harvested at day 6 of culture for cryopreservation in FCS/10 % DMSO at −150 °C. After thawing and washing, these cells can be cultured in the presence of GMCSF for 2–3 days to generate GMCSF-DCs for the suppression assay.

9. An aliquot of GMCSF-DCs should be analyzed by flow cytometry for the expression of CD11c, MHC class II, and CD86. More than 70 % of the cells should express CD11c. Among CD11c$^{+}$ cells, not more than 30 % should have an MHC class II$^{hi}$CD86$^{hi}$ mature phenotype.
10. We typically use the indicated Invitrogen kits. However, other methods for the isolation of T cells may be used. We strongly recommend the use of negative T cell isolation because the binding of anti-CD4 antibodies may inhibit effector T cell functions. Mayer et al. J Autoimmun 2013 (PMID: 24055067) Mayer et al. J Autoimmun 2014 (PMID: 24075450).
11. Tregs may be purified from WT mice by MACS.
12. To reduce sorting time (especially if more DEREG mice are processed), CD4$^{+}$ T cells can be enriched prior to sorting following Subheading 3.2 (**steps 1–6**).
13. Here, only ratios of 1:1 and 1:5 (Tregs:Tresp) are used. However, it is generally recommended to test multiple ratios (e.g., 1:1, 1:2, 1:5, 1:10, 1:20).
14. Regularly monitor the cells using a light microscope. T cell activation and the formation of proliferation clusters should be easily noticed in the positive control wells of a successful assay. If the cells proliferate extensively and the medium turns yellow, the assay may be already analyzed earlier (e.g. on day 4).
15. With the configuration of our LSRII cytometer, CFSE and PE have almost no spectral overlap. However, other flow cytometers may require careful compensation of the two channels. This can be avoided by using anti-CD45.1-eFluor450 instead of the PE conjugate.
16. Using the described panel, only minimal compensation is necessary. Most attention is required for CFSE vs. PE/PI/EMA (depending on the cytometer, *see* **Note 15**) and PE vs. PI/EMA.
17. CFSE fluorescence can affect the PI/EMA channels if not properly compensated.
18. The CD4$^{+}$CD45.1$^{-}$ cells are Tregs; gating on these may provide additional information (e.g., to detect the stability of Foxp3/eGFP expression). Moreover, additional antibodies (e.g., directed against activation markers) can be included in the analyses.

## Acknowledgement

We thank Maxine Swallow, Friederike Kruse, Melanie Gohmert, Martina Thiele, and Maike Hegemann for expert technical assistance and Dr. Katharina Lahl, Catharina Arnold Schrauf, Christina Hesse, and Venkateswaran Ganesh for critical reading of the manuscript. C.T.M. was supported by the German National Academic

Foundation. We would further like to thank the Cell Sorting Core Facility of the Hannover Medical School supported in part by the Braukmann-Wittenberg-Herz-Stiftung and Deutsche Forschungsgemeinschaft.

## References

1. Mayer CT, Berod L, Sparwasser T (2012) Layers of dendritic cell-mediated T cell tolerance, their regulation and the prevention of autoimmunity. Front Immunol 3:183. doi:10.3389/fimmu.2012.00183
2. Berod L, Puttur F, Huehn J, Sparwasser T (2012) Tregs in infection and vaccinology: heroes or traitors? Microb Biotechnol 5(2):260–269. doi:10.1111/j.1751-7915.2011.00299.x
3. Klages K, Mayer CT, Lahl K, Loddenkemper C, Teng MW, Ngiow SF, Smyth MJ, Hamann A, Huehn J, Sparwasser T (2010) Selective depletion of Foxp3+ regulatory T cells improves effective therapeutic vaccination against established melanoma. Cancer Res 70(20):7788–7799. doi:10.1158/0008-5472.CAN-10-1736, 0008-5472.CAN-10-1736 [pii]
4. Takahashi T, Kuniyasu Y, Toda M, Sakaguchi N, Itoh M, Iwata M, Shimizu J, Sakaguchi S (1998) Immunologic self-tolerance maintained by CD25+CD4+ naturally anergic and suppressive T cells: induction of autoimmune disease by breaking their anergic/suppressive state. Int Immunol 10(12):1969–1980
5. Thornton AM, Shevach EM (1998) CD4+CD25+ immunoregulatory T cells suppress polyclonal T cell activation in vitro by inhibiting interleukin 2 production. J Exp Med 188(2):287–296
6. Lahl K, Loddenkemper C, Drouin C, Freyer J, Arnason J, Eberl G, Hamann A, Wagner H, Huehn J, Sparwasser T (2007) Selective depletion of Foxp3+ regulatory T cells induces a scurfy-like disease. J Exp Med 204(1):57–63. doi:10.1084/jem.20061852, jem.20061852 [pii]
7. Kim J, Lahl K, Hori S, Loddenkemper C, Chaudhry A, deRoos P, Rudensky A, Sparwasser T (2009) Cutting edge: depletion of Foxp3+ cells leads to induction of autoimmunity by specific ablation of regulatory T cells in genetically targeted mice. J Immunol 183(12):7631–7634. doi:10.4049/jimmunol.0804308, jimmunol.0804308 [pii]
8. Mayer CT, Kuhl AA, Loddenkemper C, Sparwasser T (2012) Lack of Foxp3+ macrophages in both untreated and B16 melanoma-bearing mice. Blood 119(5):1314–1315. doi:10.1182/blood-2011-11-392266, 119/5/1314 [pii]
9. Mayer CT, Floess S, Baru AM, Lahl K, Huehn J, Sparwasser T (2011) CD8+ Foxp3+ T cells share developmental and phenotypic features with classical CD4+ Foxp3+ regulatory T cells but lack potent suppressive activity. Eur J Immunol 41(3):716–725. doi:10.1002/eji.201040913
10. Baru AM, Untucht C, Ganesh V, Hesse C, Mayer CT, Sparwasser T (2012) Optimal isolation of functional Foxp3+ induced regulatory T cells using DEREG mice. PLoS One 7(9):e44760. doi:10.1371/journal.pone.0044760
11. Zal T, Volkmann A, Stockinger B (1994) Mechanisms of tolerance induction in major histocompatibility complex class II-restricted T cells specific for a blood-borne self-antigen. J Exp Med 180(6):2089–2099
12. Lutz MB, Kukutsch N, Ogilvie AL, Rossner S, Koch F, Romani N, Schuler G (1999) An advanced culture method for generating large quantities of highly pure dendritic cells from mouse bone marrow. J Immunol Methods 223(1):77–92

# Chapter 10

# In Vitro Generation of Microbe-Specific Human Th17 Cells

Julia M. Braun and Christina E. Zielinski

## Abstract

Th17 cells represent a T helper cell subset with major implications for the pathogenesis of autoimmune diseases and the clearance of extracellular bacteria and fungi. The in vitro generation of human Th17 cells has been subject to many debates concerning the minimal cytokine requirements for IL-17 induction. This is partly due to the low Th17 cell priming efficiencies that have been reported so far for human as compared to murine T cells. In addition, human T helper cell priming is primarily performed using polyclonal stimulation even though it has recently been reported that cytokine requirements for the generation of Th17 cells may differ depending on the microbial antigen specificities of naïve T cells. Here, we present a detailed procedure on how to efficiently generate microbe-specific Th17 cells from naïve T helper cells.

**Key words** T cells, Th17 cells, *Candida albicans*

## 1 Introduction

IL-17-producing T cells have been described in settings of chronic inflammation and infection about 15 years prior [1] to their recognition as a separate T helper cell lineage, the Th17 cell subset [2, 3]. In recent years, the characterization of Th17 cells has progressed at a high pace. In particular, the differentiation requirements of Th17 cells have been subject to intense investigations and have also yielded controversies with respect to the minimal cytokine requirements for IL-17 induction as well as the IL-17-promoting versus -suppressive role of TGF-β. We now have learned that different priming requirements for Th17 cells coexist in both mice and humans and that they entail different functional phenotypes [4]. The combination of TGF-β and IL-6 generates nonpathogenic Th17 cells whereas the combination of IL-1β, IL-6, and IL-23 leads to Th17 cells with pro-inflammatory functions in mice [5]. In humans, the poor efficiency in the induction of IL-17-producing T cells from naïve $CD4^+$ T cell precursors has culminated in many different reports on the essential cytokine requirements for Th17 cell differentiation. Recently, the existence of two subsets of Th17

Ari Waisman and Burkhard Becher (eds.), *T-Helper Cells: Methods and Protocols*, Methods in Molecular Biology, vol. 1193, DOI 10.1007/978-1-4939-1212-4_10, © Springer Science+Business Media New York 2014

cells has also been reported in humans [6]. The generation of pro- versus anti-inflammatory Th17 cells is contingent on the presence of IL-1β, which suppresses IL-10 and induces IFN-γ expression [6]. Interestingly, the requirement for IL-1β for the generation of human Th17 cells is determined by the antigen specificity of naïve T helper cells. The generation of *C. albicans*-specific Th17 cells is dependent on IL-1β, whereas IL-6 and IL-23 suffice for the generation of *S. aureus*-specific Th17 cells [6]. In contrast to polyclonal Th17 cell generation protocols, the generation of pathogen-specific Th17 cells yields high levels of IL-17. This allows a detailed dissection of Th17 cell priming requirements in response to different microbes and further characterization of the functional characteristics of the ensuing antigen-specific Th17 cells [7]. In Subheading 3 the detailed procedure for the generation of microbe-specific human Th17 cells from naïve $CD4^+$ T cell precursors is presented.

## 2 Materials

### 2.1 Cell Culture

1. Complete culture medium: Supplement RPMI 1640 medium with 5 % human serum (pooled from 50 to 100 donors), 1 % L-glutamine, 1 % sodium pyruvate, 1 % nonessential amino acids, 0.1 % β-mercaptoethanol, as well as 1 % penicillin/streptomycin. Store at 4 °C for max. 2 weeks.
2. Wash buffer: Supplement RPMI 1640 containing 25 mM HEPES with 0.5 % human serum. Store at 4 °C.
3. MACS buffer: Supplement PBS with 5 % human serum and 2 mM EDTA. Store at 4 °C.
4. FACS buffer: Supplement Dulbecco's PBS with 1 % fetal cow serum (FCS) and 0.01 % $NaN_3$. Store at 4 °C.
5. 96-Well microtiter polystyrene plates (preferably from Costar).
6. Basic cell culture equipment: Incubator, laminar flow hood.

### 2.2 Monocyte Isolation

1. Ficoll-Hypaque Plus (GE Healthcare) (*see* **Note 1**).
2. Magnetic cell separator (Miltenyi Biotec).
3. Human CD14 MicroBeads (Miltenyi Biotec).
4. 25 and 50 mL polypropylene conical tubes (for cell collection, cell washing, incubation with antibodies, cell resting).

### 2.3 T Cell Isolation

1. Ficoll-Hypaque Plus (GE Healthcare).
2. Human CD4 MACS MicroBeads (Miltenyi Biotec).
3. Naïve T cell sorting: Anti-CD45RO-Fitc (Immunotech), anti-CD25-Fitc (Immunotech), anti-CD8-Fitc (Immunotech), anti-CCR7 (150503, R&D Systems), biotinylated anti-IgG2a

(Southern Biotech), Streptavidin-Pacific blue (Molecular Probes; Invitrogen).

4. Flow cytometer (i.e., FACSCanto, BD Biosciences).

### 2.4 Intracellular Cytokine Staining

1. Ionomycin (Sigma-Aldrich, 1 μg/mL final concentration).
2. Phorbol-12-myristate-13-acetate (PMA) (Sigma-Aldrich, $2 \times 10^{-7}$ final concentration).
3. Brefeldin A (BFA) (Sigma-Aldrich, 10 μg/mL final concentration).
4. BD Cytofix/Cytoperm™ Kit (BD Biosciences).
5. Cell sorter (i.e., FACSAria, BD Biosciences).

### 2.5 T Cell Labeling with Carboxy-fluorescein Succinimidyl Ester (CFSE)

1. Dulbecco's PBS.
2. CFSE solution (final concentration 0.5 μM) (*see* **Note 2**).

## 3 Methods

### 3.1 Isolation of Monocytes

1. Isolate PBMC by density centrifugation using Ficoll-Hypaque (GE Healthcare) according to standard protocols (*see* **Note 1**).
2. Wash 1× with MACS buffer.
3. Stain PBMC for 30 min on ice with CD14 MicroBeads (Miltenyi Biotec) in MACS buffer according to the manufacturer's protocol.
4. Perform positive selection of $CD14^+$ monocytes by loading the cell suspension onto a MACS column placed in the magnetic field of a MACS Separator (*see* **Note 3**).
5. Wash with 3× 3 mL MACS buffer.
6. Elute the magnetically retained $CD14^+$ cells by removing the MACS columns from the magnetic field and flushing them with 2× 3 mL MACS buffer using the provided plunger.
7. Keep the negative fraction containing T cells for later use (i.e., isolation of naïve T helper cells).
8. Spin down the positive cell fraction ($CD14^+$ cells). Resuspend in 5 mL wash buffer and let the cells rest on ice until needed for incubation with pathogens or their respective lysates.
9. Freeze down monocytes for later use (i.e., for validation of microbial antigen specificity of in vitro-generated Th17 cells).

### 3.2 Incubation of Monocytes with Pathogens

1. Irradiate monocytes with 45 Gy to prevent the selective outgrowth of potentially contaminating memory T helper cells during T cell priming experiments (*see* **Note 4**).

2. Wash irradiated monocytes 2× with wash buffer immediately after irradiation.
3. Let irradiated monocytes rest for at least 3 h on ice.
4. Wash rested irradiated monocytes with wash buffer once.
5. Spin down monocytes and resuspend them in complete culture medium (*see* **Note 5**).
6. Distribute 80 μL of monocyte cell suspension into round-bottom wells of 96-well microtiter plates.
7. Add 20 μL of your microbial lysate of choice or suspension of intact microbes on top of the monocyte culture (*see* **Note 6**).
8. Keep monocyte cultures without any microbial antigens as one of the negative controls for the co-culture experiments.
9. Incubate/pulse monocytes for 3 h with the microbial lysates or intact microbe suspensions (*see* **Note 7**).
10. During the 3-h incubation/pulsing period proceed with the sorting and CFSE labeling of naïve T helper cells (*see* Subheading 3.3).
11. After 3 h of incubation, monocytes in control cultures may be analyzed for cell viability and activation marker upregulation. If *C. albicans* is used, the yeast particles will not be visible anymore by conventional light microscopy.

### 3.3 Isolation of Naïve Human T Helper Cells

1. Take the negative fraction of PBMC after $CD14^+$ depletion by MACS separation and run the CD14-depleted PBMC through a fresh MACS column to deplete any remaining MACS beads.
2. Collect the $CD14^-$ PBMC after depletion of MACS MicroBeads.
3. Spin down the cell suspension and stain with CD4 MACS MicroBeads (Miltenyi Biotec) diluted in 2 mL MACS buffer for 30 min on ice according to the manufacturer's protocol.
4. Perform a positive selection of $CD4^+$ cells (*see* Subheading 3.1). Elute the magnetically retained $CD4^+$ cells with 2× 3 mL MACS buffer. Discard the negative fraction.
5. Spin down the cell suspension and resuspend in MACS buffer. Stain cells with monoclonal antibodies for CD45RO, CD8, CD25, and CCR7. Incubate on ice for 30 min (*see* **Note 8**).
6. Isolate naïve T helper cells with a cell sorter as $CD45RO^-$, $CD8^-$, $CD25^-$, and $CCR7^+$ cells into FACS tubes filled with wash buffer (Fig. 1).
7. Spin down cell suspension, resuspend with wash buffer, and let the cells rest for at least 30 min on ice before proceeding to CSFE labeling (*see* **Note 9**).

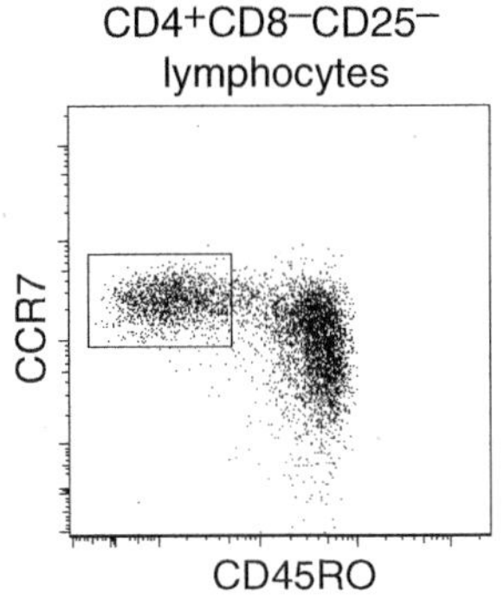


**Fig. 1** Sorting of naïve T helper cells

### 3.4 CFSE Labeling of Naïve T Helper Cells

1. Let cell suspension slowly acquire room temperature.
2. Wash cells 2× with PBS at room temperature.
3. Resuspend cells in 1 mL PBS and label cells with CFSE (carboxyfluorescein succinimidyl ester) by adding 1 mL of 1 μM CFSE solution (final concentration 0.5 μM; final volume 2 mL) (*see* **Note 9**).
4. Incubate cells with CFSE solution in the dark for 8 min with gentle shaking at room temperature.
5. Add complete culture medium dropwise until the tube is filled up and spin cells down at 4 °C (*see* **Note 9**).
6. Wash 3× with complete culture medium at 4 °C to quench CSFE.
7. Resuspend cells in wash buffer and let cells rest for 30–60 min on ice in wash buffer before co-culture with microbe pulsed monocytes.

### 3.5 Co-culture of Microbe-Pulsed Monocytes with Naïve T Helper Cells

1. After pulsing monocytes for 3 h, add 100 μL of CFSE-labeled naïve T helper cells at a concentration of 500,000/mL in complete medium on top of microbe-pulsed monocytes (*see* **Note 10**).
2. Keep cultures with monocytes alone, T cells alone, as well as co-cultures in the absence of microbial antigens as controls (*see* **Note 11**).
3. After 9–12 days of culture, FACS analysis in combination with intracellular cytokine staining can be performed to determine the cytokine profile of the responding $CFSE^{low}$ T cell population (*see* **Note 12**).

### 3.6 FACS Analysis

1. Harvest cells on days 9–12 and perform intracellular cytokine staining following 5-h PMA and ionomycin restimulation in the presence of brefeldin A for the last 2.5 h.

2. For fixation and permeabilization we recommend following the manufacturer's instructions of the BD Cytofix/Cytoperm™ Kit (BD Biosciences) (*see* **Notes 13** and **14**).

### *3.7 Validation of Antigen Specificity of In Vitro-Primed T Helper Cells*

1. Isolate CFSE-negative T cells on days 9–12 by cell sorting.
2. Let the cells rest for 5–7 days in IL-2-containing complete medium (50 IU/mL IL-2).
3. Spin cells down and perform T cell cloning by limiting dilution as described previously using phytohemagglutinin (PHA, 1 μg/mL, Remel), irradiated allogeneic feeder cells (45 Gy), and complete media supplemented with 500 IU/mL IL-2 [8].
4. After T cell clones reach the resting state (12–20 days after stimulation) restimulate them with autologous monocytes (frozen samples) pulsed with the microbes of interest as described above (T cell:monocyte ratio 2:1–4:1).
5. Keep control cultures with T cells and monocytes that have not been pulsed with microbial antigens.
6. After 48 h add $^3$H-thymidine.
7. After another 16 h determine proliferation by $^3$H-thymidine incorporation using a scintillation counter according to standard protocols (*see* **Note 15**). Correlate the polarization of in vitro-generated human T helper cells with the ex vivo polarization pattern of antigen-specific T helper cells. This indicates that the in vitro Th17 polarization conditions described herein match the in vivo situation (*see* **Note 16**).

## 4 Notes

1. This Ficoll is well suited for the isolation of human monocytes compared to several other tested products that might unspecifically activate monocytes and therefore cause artifacts in antigen-specific T cell priming.
2. Prepare always freshly from 5 mM stock solution.
3. Use a 30 μm nylon mesh filter to avoid clumps in the MACS columns.
4. The irradiation dose may differ depending on the gamma irradiator used.
5. If the microbe of choice for T cell priming is *C. albicans*, resuspend monocytes at a concentration of 312,500 cells/mL. *C. albicans* will induce the generation of Th17 cells. Other microbes are expected to have different polarization effects.
6. The final concentration of those microbial antigens needs to be determined by titration using cell viability (apoptosis and cell death) and activation markers like CD80 and CD86 as readout.

If *C. albicans* is used, the optimal ratio is three *C. albicans* yeast particles per monocyte. After about 20–30 min, it is possible to visualize the internalization of maximal three round yeast particles within individual monocytes by conventional light microscopy. The concentration will also affect the strength of T cell activation.

7. The optimum duration of this co-incubation may differ depending on the microbial species or the preparation used. For intact heat-inactivated *C. albicans*, 3 h of incubation leads to a cytokine milieu that optimally favors the generation of Th17 cells from naïve T helper cell precursors.
8. For CCR7 labeling we recommend successive staining with CCR7, followed by biotinylated anti-IgG2a and streptavidin-Pacific blue.
9. CSFE is highly toxic for cells. Although other alternative CFSE labeling protocols for human T cells are available we recommend our optimized protocol. Protocols for human and mouse CFSE labeling differ and should not be interchanged.
10. For *C. albicans*-pulsed monocytes the optimum T cell-to-monocyte ratio range is 2:1–4:1. For other microbes or their respective lysates optimum ratio ranges should be titrated to determine optimum proliferative responses.
11. You may also stimulate naïve T helper cells polyclonally with anti-CD3 and anti-CD28 as a control.
12. As the frequency of antigen-specific T cells in the naïve T cell repertoire is very low, the proliferating antigen-responsive T cell population will be oligoclonal. After about 5–7 days of culture these few cells will significantly expand giving rise to a bigger population of effector T cells. After 5–7 days, IL-2 levels increase and might start inducing antigen-nonspecific proliferation of CFSE-negative cells. They can easily be excluded from the analysis based on CFSE high versus low staining.
13. Monocytes can be excluded based on $CD14^+$ surface staining but after the 9–12-day culture period they should not be detectable anymore.
14. If T cell priming is performed using *C. albicans*-pulsed monocytes, naïve T helper cells will polarize into IL-17 and IFN-γ coproducing effector T cells that are unable to produce IL-10 upon restimulation.
15. The readout is counts per minute (cpm). Cultures can be scored positive when the stimulation index is bigger than 5 and when the delta value (cpm in response to antigen-pulsed monocytes – cpm in response to unpulsed monocytes) exceeds $3 \times 10^3$ cpm. Control cultures set up in the absence of microbial antigens are expected to show counts below $10^3$ cpm, which is

consistent with lack of reactivity to autologous monocytes and human serum components. We expect between 80 and 90 % of all tested clones to respond in this microbial recall assay.

16. In the case of *C. albicans*, ex vivo-isolated memory Th17 cells ($CCR6^+CCR4^+CXCR3^-CD45RA^-CD3^+CD4^+$), but not Th1 ($CCR6^-CCR4^-CXCR3^+CD45RA^-CD3^+CD4^+$) and Th2 ($CCR6^-CCR4^+CXCR3^-CD45RA^-CD3^+CD4^+$) cells, preferentially proliferate in recall assays using *C. albicans*-pulsed monocytes (5-day stimulation period).

## Acknowledgements

This work has been supported by the Deutsche Forschungsgemeinschaft (SFB650 and DFG ZI-1262) and the Celgene Award and the Else Kröner-Fresenius Foundation for Innovation and Immunology Research into Dermatological Diseases. We thank Federica Sallusto for valuable suggestions for establishing the presented method.

### References

1. Annunziato F, Cosmi L, Liotta F, Maggi E, Romagnani S (2012) Trends Immunol 33: 505–512
2. Kotake S, Udagawa N, Takahashi N, Matsuzaki K, Itoh K, Ishiyama S, Saito S, Inoue K, Kamatani N, Gillespie MT, Martin TJ, Suda T (1999) J Clin Invest 103:1345–1352
3. Infante-Duarte C, Horton HF, Byrne MC, Kamradt T (2000) J Immunol 165: 6107–6115
4. Sallusto F, Zielinski CE, Lanzavecchia A (2012) Eur J Immunol 42:2215–2220
5. Ghoreschi K, Laurence A, Yang XP, Tato CM, McGeachy MJ, Konkel JE, Ramos HL, Wei L, Davidson TS, Bouladoux N, Grainger JR, Chen Q, Kanno Y, Watford WT, Sun HW, Eberl G, Shevach EM, Belkaid Y, Cua DJ, Chen W, O'Shea JJ (2010) Nature 467:967–971
6. Zielinski CE, Mele F, Aschenbrenner D, Jarrossay D, Ronchi F, Gattorno M, Monticelli S, Lanzavecchia A, Sallusto F (2012) Nature 484:514–518
7. Zielinski CE, Corti D, Mele F, Pinto D, Lanzavecchia A, Sallusto F (2011) Immunol Rev 240:40–51
8. Messi M, Giacchetto I, Nagata K, Lanzavecchia A, Natoli G, Sallusto F (2003) Nat Immunol 4:78–86

# Chapter 11

# In Vitro Polarization of T-Helper Cells

Julie Rumble and Benjamin M. Segal

## Abstract

In vitro polarization of $CD4^+$ T cells along distinct T-helper (Th) lineages is critical for defining the factors and properties that determine the differentiation, stability, and effector functions of each Th subset. Furthermore, polarized cells can be transferred into naïve syngeneic mice to investigate their trafficking patterns and pathological or therapeutic roles in the setting of infection, autoimmunity, and neoplasia. In this chapter, we describe methods for generating and characterizing a spectrum of $CD4^+$ Th cell lines in vitro. Protocols are provided that use naïve wild-type or T cell receptor (TCR) transgenic CD4+ T cells, or a polyclonal population of primed CD4+ T cells from immunized mice.

**Key words** T-helper cells, CD4+ T cells, Lymphocytes, Cytokines, Polarization

## 1 Introduction

The fact that $CD4^+$ T helper cells are heterogenous and can be categorized into subsets based on cytokine profiling was originally recognized by Mosmann and Coffman [1]. A series of subsequent studies in animal models showed that Th1 and Th2 cells naturally arise in vivo in the setting of infection and neoplasia as well as allergy and autoimmune disease [2–4]. Furthermore, the Th bias of an immune response can have profound implications regarding clinical outcomes [5–7].

Since Mosmann and Coffman's seminal study that characterized Th1 and Th2 clones, a host of distinct Th lineages have been identified. Each of these lineages arises as a consequence of a unique differentiation program, driven by specific polarizing cytokines and transcription factors, and subserves specialized functions. Some Th subsets are particularly effective at guiding protective immune responses against specific classes of pathogens, but have also been implicated in autoimmune or allergic pathogenesis. The characteristics of Th subsets, as currently defined, are summarized in Table 1.

The ability to polarize CD4 T helper (Th) cells in vitro towards distinct lineages can be a powerful tool for analyzing the function

Ari Waisman and Burkhard Becher (eds.), *T-Helper Cells: Methods and Protocols*, Methods in Molecular Biology, vol. 1193, DOI 10.1007/978-1-4939-1212-4_11, © Springer Science+Business Media New York 2014

**Table 1**
**Characteristics of CD4+ Th cell subsets**

| | Transcription factor | Signature cytokine | Polarizing cytokines | In vivo functions |
|---|---|---|---|---|
| Th1 [17] | T-bet | IFN-γ | IL-12 | Clearance of intracellular bacteria and viruses, antitumor immunity; organ-specific autoimmunity; monocyte activation and recruitment |
| Th2 [17] | GATA3 | IL-4 | IL-4 | Clearance of parasitic helminths; allergic responses; eosinophilia |
| Th17 [18] | RORγt | IL-17 | TGF-β, IL-6, IL-23 | Clearance of extracellular bacteria; organ-specific autoimmunity; neutrophil mobilization and chemotaxis |
| Th9 [19, 20] | STAT6, GATA3 | IL-9 | TGF-β, IL4 | Clearance of parasites; asthma; mast cell proliferation and activation |
| Th22 [21] | AhR, T-bet | IL-22 | IL-6, TNF | Induction of epidermal immune responses; tissue remodeling |
| Treg [22] | FoxP3 | | TGF-β | Regulation of proinflammatory immune responses |
| Tfh [23] | Bcl6 | IL-21 | IL-6, IL-21 | B cell help; germinal center maintenance |

of Th subsets in vivo. Animal models of autoimmune diseases as well as protective immune responses (against infections and tumors) have been developed based on the adoptive transfer of highly polarized Th cell lines or clones [8–11].

In some cases, naïve ($CD44^{-}CD25^{-}CD62L^{+}$) $CD4^{+}$ T cells are isolated from the lymph nodes and/or spleens of T cell receptor transgenic donors and stimulated with antigen and polarizing cocktails prior to transfer [12]. In other instances, CD4+ T cells obtained from immunized (non-TCR transgenic) mice are subjected to similar protocols [13]. In the latter case, the T cell lines thus generated are polyclonal and heterogeneous; however Th cells reactive against the intended antigen are preferentially selected and expanded. Since donor mice are often primed with antigen in combination with complete Freund's adjuvant (CFA), the Mycobacterial components contained in the adjuvant could promote the initial in vivo priming towards Th1 or Th17 lineages. In order to avoid such a bias, an alternative approach is to prime mice with incomplete Freund's adjuvant (IFA) [14, 15]. The use of alum as an adjuvant can also be used to favor Th2 responses [16].

## 2 Materials

1. Complete media (CM): RPMI 1640, 10 % FBS, 55 mM beta-mercaptoethanol, 1 mM sodium pyruvate, 1× NEAA, 2 mM L-glutamine, 1× Pen/Strep, 12.5 mM Hepes.
2. Consumables: 70 mm mesh screens, 24-well tissue culture treated plates, 3 ml syringes.
3. CD4+ T cell purification: MACS Miltenyi kit: mouse CD4+ CD62L$^{hi}$ (#130-093-227) or flow sorter (*see* **Note 1**) and antibodies to CD4 (L3T4), CD62L (MEL-14), and CD25 (PC61).
4. In vitro Culture: Antigen of choice (peptide or purified protein); Recombinant mouse cytokines: IL-12, IFN-γ, IL-4, TGF-β, IL-6, IL-21, IL-23 (*see* **Note 2**); Monoclonal antibodies: anti-CD3 (145-2C11), anti-CD28 (37.51), anti-IL-4 (clone A11B11), anti-IFN-γ (Xμg1.2), anti-TGF-β (1D11), anti-IL-12 (C17.8).
5. FACS staining to confirm successful polarization: 100 μg/ml phorbol myristate acid (PMA) in 100 % ethanol, 5 μg/ml ionomycin in DMSO, 2 μg/ml Brefeldin A in DMSO, FACS buffer: PBS, 2 % FBS, 0.5 μg/ml Fc block (clone 2.4G2), 4 % paraformaldehyde (PFA) in PBS, 0.5 % saponin from quillaja bark in FACS buffer, Transcription Factor Buffer Set (BD Pharmingen cat # 562574, *see* **Note 8**).
6. Monoclonal antibodies for flow cytometric analysis: anti-CD3 (145-2C11), anti-CD4 (L3T4), anti-IFN-γ (Xμg1.2), anti-T-bet (ebio4b10), anti-IL-4 (BVD6-24G2), anti-IL-13 (ebio1316H), anti-GATA-3 (TWAJ), anti-IL-17 (TC11-18H10), anti-RORγt (AFJKS-9), anti-CD25 (PC61.5), anti-FoxP3 (NRRF-30), anti-IL-9 (RM9A4), anti-IL10 (JES5-16E3), anti-B220 (RA3-6B2), anti-CXCR5 (SPRCL5), anti-PD-1 (J43), anti-BCL-6 (μgI191E), anti-ICOS (C398.4A), anti-IL-22 (IL22JOP), anti-TNF (MP6-XT22).

## 3 Methods

### 3.1 Polarization of Naïve TCR Transgenic CD4+ T Cells (See Note 3)

1. For this protocol, TCR-transgenic mice are used as a source of CD4+ T cells and syngeneic wild-type mice are used as a source of antigen presenting cells (APC). Euthanize mice from each group, spray fur with 70 % ethanol, and remove spleens (keeping transgenic separate from non-transgenic cells).
2. Place spleens in a conical tube filled with complete media (CM) on ice. The remaining steps should be performed in a tissue culture hood to maintain antiseptic conditions.

3. Separate splenocytes into a single cell suspension by passage through a 70 mm screen into a 50 ml conical tube. (Use the plunger from a 3 ml syringe to force cells through the screen. Apply CM over the screen several times to wash the cells through).
4. Fill tube with CM and spin at $500 \times g$, 5 min, 4 °C.
5. Decant supernatant and add 5 ml ACK lysis buffer Vortex.
6. Incubate at room temperature (RT) for 2–3 min, then resuspend cells in 25 ml fresh CM, and spin again.
7. Aspirate supernatant and resuspend the pellet in 10 ml CM. Count live cells using a hemocytometer by trypan blue exclusion.
8. TCR transgenic splenocytes only: Isolate CD62L+CD4+ naïve T cells using MACS Miltenyi beads following the manufacturer's instructions (*see* **Note 2**).
9. Wild-type splenocytes only: irradiate with 30 Gy source. These cells will be referred to as APCs hereafter.
10. Spin cells down and resuspend in CM. Combine T-depleted APCs and naïve TCR transgenic cells in CM at a 5:1 ratio. Add media to a final concentration of $10 \times 10^6$ total cells/ml. Aliquot 1 ml of cell suspension per well in 24 well plates.
11. Dilute antigenic peptide, polarizing cytokines, and neutralizing antibodies in CM to twice their final concentrations. The concentration of antigen varies based on the model. The *final* concentration of polarizing cytokines and neutralizing antibodies for each lineage should be as follows:
    (a) Th1: IL-12 (5 ng/ml), IFN-γ (2 ng/ml), anti-IL-4 (10 μg/ml)
    (b) Th2: IL-4 (20 ng/ml), anti-IFN-γ (10 μg/ml)
    (c) Th17: TGF-β (5 ng/ml), IL-6 (20 ng/ml), anti-IFN-γ (10 μg/ml), anti-IL4 (10 μg/ml)
    (d) Treg: TGF-β (5 ng/ml)
    (e) Th9: TGF-β (5 ng/ml), IL-4 (20 ng/ml)
    (f) Tfh: IL-6 (100 ng/ml), IL-21 (50 ng/ml), anti-TGF-β (20 μg/ml), anti-IFN-γ (10 μg/ml), anti-IL-4 (10 μg/ml), anti-IL-12 (10 μg/ml)
    (g) Th22: IL-6 (100 ng/ml), IL-23 (20 ng/ml), anti-TGF-β (20 μg/ml), anti-IFN-γ (10 μg/ml)
12. Add 1 ml of the peptide/polarizing cocktail mixture to each well.
13. Incubate cells at 37 °C for 4–5 days (*see* **Note 4**).

### 3.2 Polarization of Primed CD4+ T Cells

1. Perform under aseptic conditions: Prepare emulsion of antigen in CFA, IFA, or alum, depending on experimental needs (*see* **Note 5**).

(a) Suspend peptide antigen in PBS to a concentration of 2 μg/ml.

(b) Attach two glass syringes to a three-way stopcock.

(c) Add suspended peptide and CFA to syringes at a 1:1 mixture of aqueous solution: CFA (*see* **Note 6**).

(d) Emulsify by sliding syringe plungers back and forth while syringes are partially submerged in ice, until well mixed.

(e) Test emulsion periodically be applying a drop to PBS in a small petri dish. The emulsion is ready when the droplet stays intact rather than breaks apart and dissolves.

(f) Anesthetize mice and inject 0.1 ml of emulsion subcutaneously, distributed equally over 4 sites on the flanks (at shoulders and hips).

2. 10–14 days after immunization, euthanize mice, douse with 70 % ethanol and dissect inguinal, axillary, and brachial lymph nodes. Deposit nodes into a conical tube filled with complete media on ice (spleens may also be used).

   Perform the remaining steps under aseptic conditions.

3. Separate lymph nodes into a single cell suspension by passage through a 70 mm screen into a 50 ml conical tube. (Use the plunger from a 3 ml syringe to force cells through the screen. Apply CM over the screen several times to wash the cells through).

4. Fill tube with CM and spin at $500 \times g$, 5 min, 4 °C (If spleens are used, ACK lysis step is recommended; *see* Subheading 3.1, **steps 4** and **5**).

5. Count live cells via trypan blue exclusion using a hemocytometer. Resuspend cells to a concentration of $5 \times 10^6$/ml in complete media with antigen, polarization cytokines and antibodies at final concentrations as follows:

   (a) Th1: IL-12 (5 ng/ml), IFN-γ (2 ng/ml), anti-IL-4 (10 μg/ml)

   (b) Th2: IL-4 (20 ng/ml), anti-IFN-γ (10 μg/ml)

   (c) Th17: IL-23 (5 ng/ml), IL-1α (10 ng/ml), anti-IFN-γ (10 μg/ml), anti-IL4 (10 μg/ml)

   (d) Treg: TGF-β (5 ng/ml)

   (e) Th9: TGF-β (5 ng/ml), IL-4 (20 ng/ml), anti-IFN-γ (10 μg/ml)

   (f) Tfh: IL-6 (100 ng/ml), IL-21 (50 ng/ml), anti-TGF-β (20 μg/ml), anti-IFN-γ (10 μg/ml), anti-IL-4 (10 μg/ml), anti-IL-12 (10 μg/ml)

   (g) Th22: IL-6 (100 ng/ml), IL-23 (20 ng/ml), anti-TGF-β (20 μg/ml), anti-IFN-γ (10 μg/ml)

6. Culture cells in a flask (*see* **Note 7**) of the appropriate size at 37 °C, 5 % $CO_2$ for 96 h.

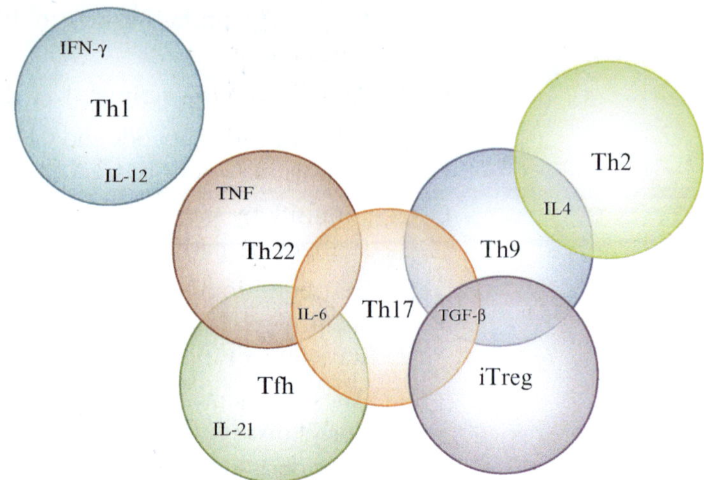


**Fig. 1** Differentiation cytokines for Th lineages

### *3.3 Assessing Degree of Polarization by Flow Cytometry (See Note 8)*

1. Transfer cells to 12 well plate at 1 ml/well.
2. Stimulate with PMA (50 ng/ml) and ionomycin (2 μg/ml) in the presence of Brefeldin A (10 μg/ml) at 37 °C for 4–6 h.
3. Transfer cells into a 15 ml conical tube, add 9 ml FACS buffer and centrifuge at $300 \times g$ for 4–5 min.
4. Resuspend pellet in FACS buffer, count and adjust concentration to $10^7$ cells/ml.
5. Aliquot 100 μl ($1 \times 10^6$ cells) in FACS tubes. Spin and resuspend in 25 μl of Fc Block diluted in FACS buffer at a concentration of 100 μg/ml. Incubate on ice for 15 min (*see* **Note 8** and Fig. 1).
6. Add 25 μl of a mastermix containing flourochrome-conjugated antibodies specific for CD4, CD3 and CD44 at appropriate concentrations. Incubate in the dark on ice for 30 min.
7. Add 200 μl FACS buffer. Centrifuge at $800 \times g$ for 5 min. Decant supernatant.
8. Wash ×2 with FACS buffer and resuspend pellet in 200 μl 4 % PFA. Incubate on ice in the dark 10 min.
9. Centrifuge at $500 \times g$ for 5 min, decant supernatant, and wash once with FACS buffer.
10. Resuspend in 200 μl of 0.5 % saponin diluted in FACS buffer. Incubate in dark at RT for 10 min.
11. Centrifuge at $500 \times g$ for 5 min, decant supernatant, and resuspend in 50 μl of mastermix containing antibodies specific for markers associated with Th subsets as follows:
    (a) Th1: *IFN*-g$^+$, *T-bet*$^+$
    (b) Th2: *IL-4*$^+$, *IL-13*$^+$, *GATA-3*$^+$

(c) Th17: *IL-17*$^+$, *ROR*$\gamma$*t*$^+$, *IFN-*$\gamma^-$

(d) Treg: **CD25**$^+$, *FoxP3*$^+$

(e) Th9: *IL-9*$^+$, *IL10*$^+$, *GATA-3*$^+$, *IL-13*$^-$

(f) Tfh: **CXCR5**$^+$, **ICOS**$^+$, **PD-1**$^+$, **B220**$^-$, *BCL-6*$^+$

(g) Th22: *IL-22*$^+$, *TNF*$^+$, *IL-17*$^-$

Incubate 30 min in the dark at RT (*see* **Note 9**).

12. Wash with saponin, resuspend in 300 ml FACS buffer, run through flow cytometer and collect $5 \times 10^4$ events or more per sample.

## 4 Notes

1. An alternative method for purifying naïve CD4+ T cells would be flow sorting for CD4$^+$ CD25$^-$ CD62L$^{hi}$ cells.
2. Storing cytokines: We purchase lyophilized cytokines and resuspend to a concentration of 100 μg/ml in PBS+0.1 % BSA. We then aliquot 10 μl into eppendorf tubes and dilute with 990 μl of complete media to obtain a working stock concentration of 1 ng/μl.
3. Naïve wild-type T cells can be polarized during polyclonal stimulation with anti-CD3. Purified naïve T cells can be plated on anti-CD3 coated plates (add 1 μg/ml anti-CD3 in PBS and incubate at 4 °C overnight, wash 3× with PBS and aliquot cells) with the addition of 2 μg/ml soluble anti-CD28. In the presence of APCs, soluble anti-CD3 can be used at a concentration of 1 μg/ml to stimulate T cells.
4. In some cases, the investigator might want to include additional cytokines to promote stabilization/final differentiation. For example, addition of recombinant IL-23 (8 ng/ml) to Th17-polarizing cultures after 2 days will generate a more highly polarized Th17 cell.
5. Incomplete Freund's adjuvant (IFA) as an alternative to CFA allows the initial priming of T cells without bias towards a particular lineage. It is recommended when the same donor cell population is used to polarize cells towards more than one lineage in parallel.
6. *See* Fig. 2 for orientation of the syringe/stopcock assembly. Remove plunger from syringe 1 for addition of reagents (stopcock in position A). Once reagents are added, pull into syringe 2 and move stopcock to position B. Replace plunger slowly into syringe 1. Move stopcock to position A and pull reagents into syringe 1. Invert assembly, move the stopcock

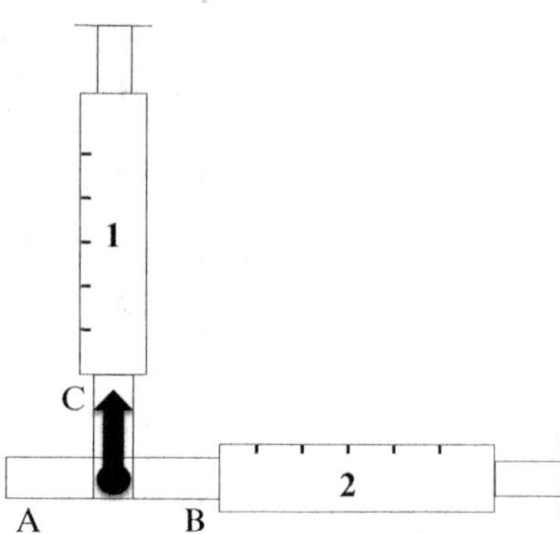


**Fig. 2** Schematic for emulsifying antigen for immunization of mice

to the negative position (opposite C), and collect remaining air bubbles at the top of syringe 1. Slowly push air out until liquid reaches the center of the stopcock and move stopcock to position A, slightly offset. Once finished emulsifying, push emulsion into syringe 2, remove syringe 1, and replace with 1 cc disposable tuberculin syringes for injecting animals. Carefully push emulsion into the new syringe. Expect to lose approximately 0.5–0.75 ml of emulsion in the stopcock.

7. Use a flask with a filtered cap or make sure the cap of the flask is not screwed on too tightly preventing adequate aeration.
8. An alternative method for determining polarization is ELISA to measure levels of cytokines, associated with different Th subsets, in culture supernatants; however, this only indicates the total amount of cytokine that has accumulated at steady state rather than the percentage of cells actually producing a cytokine of interest. In addition, this method can be not be used if the signature cytokine is a component of the polarization cocktail itself (i.e., IFN-γ in Th1 cultures).
9. We have found that for the transcription factors listed, BD Pharmingen's transcription factor buffer set (cat # 562574) works better than the PFA/saponin protocol.

## References

1. Mosmann TR, Cherwinski H, Bond MW, Giedlin MA, Coffman RL (1986) Two types of murine helper T cell clone. I. Definition according to profiles of lymphokine activities and secreted proteins. J Immunol 136:2348
2. Knutson KL, Disis ML (2005) Tumor antigen-specific T helper cells in cancer immunity and immunotherapy. Cancer Immunol Immunother 54:721
3. Infante-Duarte C, Kamradt T (1999) Th1/Th2 balance in infection. Springer Semin Immunopathol 21:317
4. Segal BM (2003) Experimental autoimmune encephalomyelitis: cytokines, effector T cells,

and antigen-presenting cells in a prototypical Th1-mediated autoimmune disease. Curr Allergy Asthma Rep 3:86

5. Heinzel FP, Sadick MD, Holaday BJ, Coffman RL, Locksley RM (1989) Reciprocal expression of interferon gamma or interleukin 4 during the resolution or progression of murine leishmaniasis. Evidence for expansion of distinct helper T cell subsets. J Exp Med 169:59
6. Lafaille JJ (1998) The role of helper T cell subsets in autoimmune diseases. Cytokine Growth Factor Rev 9:139
7. Pearson CI, McDevitt HO (1999) Redirecting Th1 and Th2 responses in autoimmune disease. Curr Top Microbiol Immunol 238:79
8. Zheng SG et al (2006) Transfer of regulatory T cells generated ex vivo modifies graft rejection through induction of tolerogenic CD4+CD25+ cells in the recipient. Int Immunol 18:279
9. Kaminuma O et al (1997) Successful transfer of late phase eosinophil infiltration in the lung by infusion of helper T cell clones. Am J Respir Cell Mol Biol 16:448
10. Muranski P, Restifo NP (2009) Adoptive immunotherapy of cancer using CD4(+) T cells. Curr Opin Immunol 21:200
11. Weber SE et al (2006) Adaptive islet-specific regulatory CD4 T cells control autoimmune diabetes and mediate the disappearance of pathogenic Th1 cells in vivo. J Immunol 176:4730
12. Lafaille JJ et al (1997) Myelin basic protein-specific T helper 2 (Th2) cells cause experimental autoimmune encephalomyelitis in immunodeficient hosts rather than protect them from the disease. J Exp Med 186:307
13. Kroenke MA, Segal BM (2011) IL-23 modulated myelin-specific T cells induce EAE via an IFNgamma driven, IL-17 independent pathway. Brain Behav Immun 25:932
14. Kroenke MA, Carlson TJ, Andjelkovic AV, Segal BM (2008) IL-12- and IL-23-modulated T cells induce distinct types of EAE based on histology, CNS chemokine profile, and response to cytokine inhibition. J Exp Med 205:1535
15. Yip HC et al (1999) Adjuvant-guided type-1 and type-2 immunity: infectious/noninfectious dichotomy defines the class of response. J Immunol 162:3942
16. Grun JL, Maurer PH (1989) Different T helper cell subsets elicited in mice utilizing two different adjuvant vehicles: the role of endogenous interleukin 1 in proliferative responses. Cell Immunol 121:134
17. Murphy KM, Reiner SL (2002) The lineage decisions of helper T cells. Nat Rev Immunol 2:933
18. Steinman L (2007) A brief history of T(H)17, the first major revision in the T(H)1/T(H)2 hypothesis of T cell-mediated tissue damage. Nat Med 13:139
19. Veldhoen M et al (2008) Transforming growth factor-beta 'reprograms' the differentiation of T helper 2 cells and promotes an interleukin 9-producing subset. Nat Immunol 9:1341
20. Dardalhon V et al (2008) IL-4 inhibits TGF-beta-induced Foxp3+ T cells and, together with TGF-beta, generates IL-9+ IL-10+ Foxp3(-) effector T cells. Nat Immunol 9:1347
21. Basu R et al (2012) Th22 cells are an important source of IL-22 for host protection against enteropathogenic bacteria. Immunity 37:1061
22. Bilate AM, Lafaille JJ (2012) Induced CD4+Foxp3+ regulatory T cells in immune tolerance. Annu Rev Immunol 30:733
23. Chtanova T et al (2004) T follicular helper cells express a distinctive transcriptional profile, reflecting their role as non-Th1/Th2 effector cells that provide help for B cells. J Immunol 173:68

# Part III

## In Vivo Models of T Cell Function

# Chapter 12

# A Method for the Generation of TCR Retrogenic Mice

**Elisa Kieback, Ellen Hilgenberg, and Simon Fillatreau**


## Abstract

Retrogenic mice provide a unique system for rapidly analyzing the function of genes in the hematopoietic system. Here, we provide a detailed protocol for the production of retrogenic mice expressing genes coding for T cell receptor (TCR) for antigen. This technology should be easy to establish in any laboratory and should allow for a rapid progress in our understanding of the functional roles of TCR repertoires in immunity.


**Key words** T cell receptor for antigen (TCR), Retrogenic mice, Retrovirus, Transduction, Transfection

## Abbreviations

| | |
|---|---|
| TCR | T cell receptor |
| ES | Embryonic stem cell |
| HSC | Hematopoietic stem cell |
| FCS | Fetal calf serum |
| PBS | Phosphate buffered saline |
| IL | Interleukin |
| SCF | Stem cell factor |
| MLV | Murine leukemia virus |
| MPSV | Myeloproliferative sarcoma virus |
| MESV | Murine embryonic stem cell virus |

## 1 Introduction

The possibility of manipulating the mouse genome offers multiple opportunities to test the function of selected genes in vivo. The production of mutant mice that can transfer the gene alteration to their progeny can be done using embryonic stem (ES) cells or oocytes, using homologous or random integration of introduced gene segments [1–3]. These technologies were the basis for many pioneering discoveries in immunology, for instance for the

Ari Waisman and Burkhard Becher (eds.), *T-Helper Cells: Methods and Protocols*, Methods in Molecular Biology, vol. 1193,
DOI 10.1007/978-1-4939-1212-4_12, © Springer Science+Business Media New York 2014

understanding of T and B lymphocyte development and selection in primary lymphoid organs [4]. Downsides of these powerful genetic approaches are that they require specialized skills, are labor-intensive, and usually necessitate at least 6 months before any genetically modified mouse can be obtained.

Compared to other physiological systems, the immune system is unique: it can be entirely replaced by immunoablation followed by transplantation of hematopoietic stem cells (HSC), which nowadays can easily be isolated, and grown in culture. Combined with the possibility of genetically modifying HSC using retroviral vectors, the feasibility of replacing the hematopoietic system through HSC transplantation has enabled the development of alternative approaches to explore the role of selected genes in immunity [5–7]. The generation of mice with a genetically engineered hematopoietic system takes only about 6–8 weeks with such approach, and the protocols for isolation and viral transduction of HSC can easily be established in individual laboratories, providing a powerful platform for the investigation of selected genes in vivo. This makes this approach suitable to test multiple genes in parallel. It is particularly well adapted to compare the properties of several T cell receptor (TCR) reacting against a chosen antigen. In comparison, it is usually difficult to generate and compare several lines of TCR transgenic mice, so that our understanding of T cell selection in the thymus is inferred in most instances from the properties of single TCR-antigens pairs. Hozumi and coworkers used this technology to express TCR chains in mouse T cells [8]. Vignali et al. later standardized this protocol [9] and showed the comparability between transgenic and retrogenic mice [10]. More than 60 different TCR have been studied in vivo using such retrogenic approach [11].

Here, we describe the protocol currently used in our laboratories to study the selection and function of antigen-reactive T cells in vivo. This method can be easily established in any laboratory, with little investment and equipment.

## 2 Materials

All cell culture reagents should be prepared and handled under sterile conditions and stored at 4 °C unless otherwise specified.

### 2.1 Production of Viral Particles

1. 6-well tissue culture plates (#353224, BD Falcon).
2. 4.5 μm pore-size filters (#16555K, Sartorius Stedim Biotech).
3. Plat-E cells [12].
4. Plat-E medium: Dulbecco's modified Eagle's medium (#61965-026, Life technologies), 10 % heat-inactivated fetal calf serum (FCS, #S0113/5, Biochrom AG) and 100 IU/ml Penicillin, Streptomycin (#15140-122, Life technologies),

puromycin (#P-7255, Sigma Aldrich), blasticidin (R210-01, Life technologies).

5. Calcium chloride buffer (2.5 M): 36.75 g calcium chloride (Sigma Aldrich), add 100 ml $H_2O$. Filter sterile and store in 500 μl aliquots at −20 °C.
6. Transfection buffer: 1.6 g NaCl, 74 mg KCl, 50 mg $Na_2HPO_4$, 1 g HEPES (all Sigma Aldrich), add 100 ml $H_2O$, pH 6.76 (exact pH and a well-calibrated pH meter are critical). Filter sterile and store at 1–3 ml aliquots at −20 °C.
7. 12 ml polystyrene tubes (#164161, Greiner).

### 2.2 HSC Isolation

1. Dissecting set: forceps with curved shanks and serrated tips (#11270-20), narrow pattern forceps (#11002-16), Iris Scissors (#14058-11, all Fine Science tools).
2. EasySep™ Mouse SCA1 Positive Selection Kit (#18756, STEMCELL Technologies).
3. EasySep™ Magnet (#18000 or #18001, STEMCELL Technologies).
4. SCA1 buffer: $Ca^{2+}$- and $Mg^{2+}$-free phosphate buffered saline (PBS, #14190136, Life technologies) with 2 % FCS (#1502, PAN Biotech) and 1 mM EDTA.
5. Stem cell medium: StemPro®-34 SFM (#10639-011, Life technologies) supplemented with 5 % FCS (#1502, PAN-Biotech), 100 IU/ml Penicillin-Streptomycin (#15150-122, Life technology), 2 mM Glutamine (#25030-081, Life technologies). Prepare 35 ml aliquots and store at −20 °C.
6. Cytokines (all PeproTech): recombinant murine interleukin-3 (IL-3) (2 μg, #213-13), recombinant murine IL-6 (10 μg, #216-16), recombinant murine stem cell factor (SCF) (10 μg, #250-03). Prepare stock solutions by diluting all cytokines in 2 ml stem cell medium and freeze at 300 μl aliquots at −20 °C. Use one of each aliquot per 30 ml of medium to yield final concentrations of 10 ng/ml for IL-3 or 50 ng/ml for IL-6 and SCF, respectively.
7. Plastic ware and other: 12 × 75 or 17 × 100 mm polystyrene round-bottom tubes (# 352054 and #352057, BD Falcon), 50 ml and 15 ml conical polypropylene tubes (#227261 and #188271, Greiner), 40 μm nylon cell strainer (BD Falcon), 1 ml syringe, 23-gauge needle, tissue culture-treated 6- and 24-well plate (#353224 and #353226, BD Falcon), counting chamber, trypan blue solution.

### 2.3 Retroviral Transduction

1. Non-tissue culture 24-well plate (#351147, BD Falcon).
2. 2 % BSA solution in PBS.
3. RetroNektin® (#T100, Takara) solution: Dilute stock solution 1:80 in PBS and freeze in 5–10 ml aliquots at −20 °C.

### 2.4 Cell Transfer

1. Radiation source ($^{137}Cs$ or X-ray).
2. Antibiotics: Dimetridazole (D4025, Sigma), Borgal 24 % (Intervet), Sirup Simplex (pharmacy). For 1 L drinking water: 1 L tap water (not distilled water!), 4 g Dimetridazole, 500 μl Borgal, 15 ml syrup. Stir well and filter sterile through 0.2 μm pore-size filter.

## 3 Methods

### 3.1 Preparation of Retroviral Supernatant

#### 3.1.1 Seeding of Packaging Cells

1. The packaging cell line Plat-E harbors stably integrated copies of murine leukemia virus (MLV) gag/pol and ecotropic MLV (MLV-eco) env genes. The retroviral particles produced by this cell line are infectious to rodent (but not human) cells and therefore require only a low biosafety level. To yield consistent cell densities and stable gag/pol and env expression Plat-E cells should always be kept in exponential growth under antibiotic selection (1 μg/ml puromycin and 10 μg/ml blasticidin) and at a low passage number.
2. Four days before transfection omit selective antibiotics.
3. About 20 h before transfection transfer $7\times10^5$–$1\times10^6$ Plat-E cells (exact cell number should be defined) in 3 ml Plat-E medium into one well of a tissue culture-treated 6-well plate to yield 60–70 % confluence on the day of transfection. Make sure cells are well distributed in the well by shaking the 6-well carefully but repeatedly when placing in the incubator. Cell density of the packaging cell line at the timepoint of transfection is critical to yield high virus titers. Keep cells at 37 °C and 5 % $CO_2$ in a humidified incubator. *See* also **Note 1**.

#### 3.1.2 Calcium Phosphate Transfection

1. Per well (using a 6-well plate) of Plat-E cells prepare 150 μl of 250 mM calcium chloride solution in distilled water containing 18 μg retroviral vector DNA (*see* **Note 2**) in a 15 ml polystyrene tube.
2. Vortex the tube constantly at medium speed and add 150 μl transfection buffer drop-wise to allow formation of homogenous calcium phosphate precipitates.
3. Incubate 15 min at room temperature (the solution should become opalescent)
4. Transfer the 300 μl precipitate-containing solution drop-wise to a well with Plat-E cells.
5. After 6 h incubation replace medium carefully with 3 ml pre-warmed Plat-E medium.

#### 3.1.3 Virus Harvest

1. Forty-eight hours after transfection harvest virus supernatant and filter through 0.45 μm pore-size filter to remove Plat-E cells that may have detached.

2. If desired, immediately provide Plat-E cells with 3 ml of fresh pre-warmed Plat-E medium for a second harvest 24 h later. Expect to harvest about 2.5 ml virus per well using a 6-well plate.
3. It is advisable to freeze aliquots of viral supernatant directly and test them before use with HSC, e.g., on a T cell line. Frozen virus can be stored several months at −80 °C. *See* also **Note 3**.

### 3.2 Isolation of HSC

#### 3.2.1 Extraction of Bone Marrow

1. Determine the number of donor mice needed. One donor mouse will typically be sufficient for reconstitution of 3–6 recipient mice, yet this might require adjustment depending on the experimental layout and mouse strain used.
2. Fill one well of a 6-well plate with 70 % ethanol and two wells with SCA1 buffer.
3. Sacrifice mice by cervical dislocation and disinfect them by submersing in 70 % ethanol.
4. Cut fur from ankle to abdomen, and separate hind leg bones from muscle by scraping with the curved forceps.
5. Remove tibia and femur from both legs, disinfect bones by submersing in 70 % ethanol for 3–5 s (critical to avoid contamination!), and wash successively in the two prepared wells with SCA1 buffer. Collect bones in a petri dish filled with SCA1 buffer on ice.
6. Place 4 ml SCA1 buffer into a $12 \times 75$ mm round-bottom tube. Firmly attach 23-gauge needle on a 1 ml syringe. Hold bone tightly with narrow pattern forceps, pierce on one end with needle, place into tube and flush the bone marrow through the bone into tube by pushing the plunger of the syringe. Flush the bone several times and then repeat with its opposing end. Use one tube per four mice (16 bones). The bones should become white as the marrow is entirely flushed through.
7. Disperse cell clumps of marrow by flushing them through the needle-syringe several times.
8. Pass cell suspension through a 40 μm nylon cell strainer, wash filter with PBS, and centrifuge for 5 min at $300 \times g$.
9. Resuspend pellet in 1 ml SCA1 buffer and count cells with trypan blue solution. Expect $0.5–1 \times 10^8$ bone marrow cells per mouse.
10. Adjust concentration to $10^8$ cells/ml, and transfer cells into a sterile $12 \times 75$ mm tube (up to $2.5 \times 10^8$ cells/tube), or a $17 \times 100$ mm tube (up to $8 \times 10^8$ cells/tube).

#### 3.2.2 Enrichment of SCA1-Positive Cells

Follow the manual provided for the Mouse SCA1 Selection Cocktail (*see* **Note 4**).

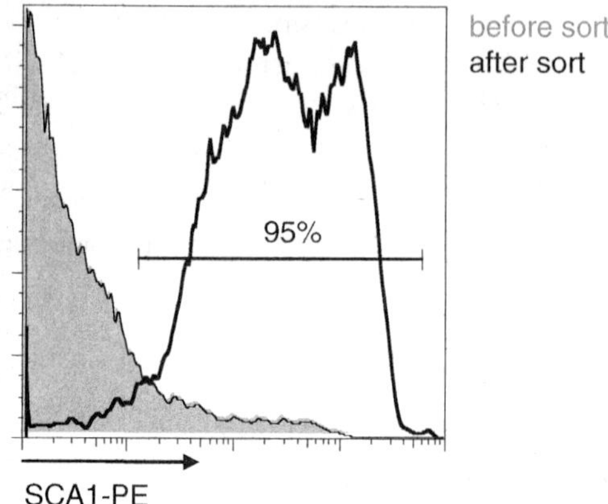


**Fig. 1** HSC can be enriched from bone marrow cells by expression of SCA1. Isolated bone marrow cells were labeled with SCA1-PE isolation reagent and analyzed by flow cytometry before and after magnetic separation

1. Add SCA1 PE labeling reagent (50 μl/ml cells) to the tube, incubate 15 min. Add PE Selection Cocktail (70 μl/ml cells), incubate another 15 min, and finally add magnetic nanoparticles (50 μl/ml cells) for 10 min (all incubation steps are performed at room temperature).
2. Fill up to the recommended volume with SCA1 buffer, and separate the SCA1-positive fraction using an EasySep® magnet for four rounds.
3. Spin cells down and resuspend the cell pellet in 5 ml stem cell medium without cytokines for washing. Centrifuge again while determining cell number. The total amount of isolated cells depends on the mouse strain used (typically $0.5–2 \times 10^6$ isolated SCA1-positive cells per mouse, less for some immunodeficient strains).
4. Resuspend cells at a concentration of $1 \times 10^6$/ml in pre-warmed stem cell medium supplemented with IL-3, IL-6, and SCF.

   If desired, the purity of SCA1-positive cells can be assessed by flow cytometry. As SCA1-positive cells are already labeled by the SCA1-PE reagent no further staining is required. *See* Fig. 1 for typical cell populations before and after enrichment.

### 3.3 Expansion and Retroviral Transduction of HSC

1. Seed $10^6$ cells in 1 ml stem cell culture medium supplemented with IL-3, IL-6, and SCF per well of a tissue-culture 24-well plate. Incubate plates at 37 °C and 5 % $CO_2$ in a humidified incubator. If possible, culture cells in a humidified chamber to disturb cells as little as possible.
2. After 3 days determine number of cells in one well to estimate total amount of cells. Per $2 \times 10^5$ cells coat one 24-well of a non-tissue culture plate with 200 μl diluted RetroNektin®

solution. Incubate at room temperature for 2 h, then replace with 200 μl 2 % BSA solution, and block for 30 min at 37 °C. Finally wash wells once with PBS, and add 500 μl of virus-containing cell supernatant per well. Spin for 2 h at 4 °C and 3,000 × *g* to promote binding of the viral particles to the plated coated with RetroNektin®.

3. Remove plates from centrifuge and let warm to 37 °C in cell culture incubator.
4. In the meantime flush HSC out of the wells, pool, and count. Spin cells down for 5 min at 250 × *g*, and resuspend in fresh stem cell medium with cytokines adjusting the concentration to $4 \times 10^5$/ml. For wild-type mice expect a slightly decreased cell number as compared to seeded cells because SCA1-positive non-HSC will have gone into apoptosis.
5. Aspirate virus-containing medium from RetroNektin® plates and seed $2 \times 10^5$ cells in 0.5 ml to each well.
6. Spin 5 min at 250 × *g* in order to facilitate contact between cells and virus.
7. Place plates into incubator at 37 °C and 5 % $CO_2$.
8. Twenty-four hours later perform the second transduction as described above.

For convenience, plates can be coated overnight with RetroNektin®. After spinoculation transfer cells 1:1 into freshly virus-coated wells (if cells have become too dense they can be expanded at this step, then prepare more virus-coated wells). Depending on cell proliferation and medium condition add additional 200–400 μl fresh stem cell medium with cytokines per well. Perform short centrifugation as above and place into incubator for 24 h, which is when cells are ready for adoptive transfer.

### 3.4 Cell Transfer

1. To allow efficient engraftment of donor HSC recipient mice need to be irradiated before transfer. Required doses should be previously defined for each radiation source and mouse strain. A typical lethal dose for wild-type animals is 900–1,200 Gy, which will allow establishing full chimerism (complete eradication of host HSC-derived cells). In contrast, a sublethal dose (around 4.5–7.2 Gy) will be sufficient for $Rag^{-/-}$ mice, other immunodeficient mice, or when only partial chimerism shall be established. Irradiation can be performed 1 h before cell transfer.
2. Twenty-four hours after second transduction flush HSC out of wells, pool, and determine cell number. Compared to their number on the day of isolation cells should have expanded four- to tenfold. If applicable, cells can be stained and analyzed by flow cytometry for transduction efficiency using marker genes.

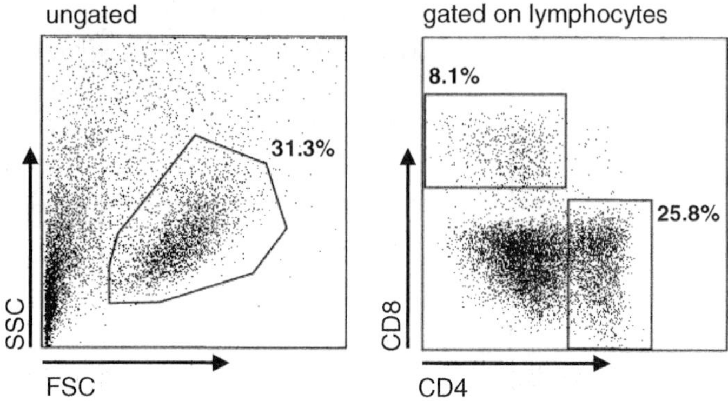


**Fig. 2** TCR-transduced HSC give rise to peripheral CD4-positive and CD8-positive T cells. HSC were isolated from bone marrow of $Rag^{-/-}$ mice and transduced with a retrovirus encoding a TCR reactive towards $MOG_{35-55}$/I-$A^b$. The genetically modified HSC were injected into irradiated $Rag^{-/-}$ recipients. Eight weeks after transfer lymph nodes of transplanted animals were isolated and stained for the presence of CD4-positive and CD8-positive T cells

Normal transduction rate ranges from 30 to 60 %. Be aware that expression of TCR genes cannot be detected in HSC emphasizing the need to use pretested virus supernatant.

3. Inject $0.5–2 \times 10^6$ HSC per mouse in 200 μl PBS into the tail vein. Transfer of $1 \times 10^5$ HSC will also lead to engraftment, but repopulation might take longer.

Depending on the pathogen status of the animal facility irradiated mice should be treated with aqueous antibiotics to prevent infections and colitis. Add Borgal or a combination of Borgal and Dimetridazole to the drinking water for at least 2 weeks, or until mice are repopulated (6–8 weeks). Successful engraftment can be detected by staining of peripheral blood T cells with TCR-specific antibodies or expression of a marker gene. Some donor-derived T cells can be found in blood as early as day 14 after transfer, but repopulation is most easily detected at about 6–8 weeks. Using a distinct combination of congenic markers such as CD45.1/2 or CD90.1/2 in donor and recipient animals allows simple discrimination between donor- and host-derived T lymphocytes. Figure 2 shows an example of reconstituted mice.

## 4 Notes

1. To yield larger quantities of virus, Plat-E cells can also be seeded into cell culture flasks or dishes. Adjust cell numbers and transfection reagents according to vessel area, and total volume.
2. Chose a retroviral vector that is well expressed in HSC, and mature T lymphocytes, and will not be silenced. Vectors

harboring a myeloproliferative sarcoma virus- (MPSV-) derived LTR, and a leader sequence of murine embryonic stem cell virus (MESV) are superior to vectors based on MLV [13]. In our hands the retroviral vector MP71-PRE [14] yields high and stable transgene expression in TCR retrogenic mice. To facilitate stoichiometric expression of the TCR alpha and TCR beta chain from the same vector use a 2A peptide [15, 16]. Derived from Picornaviruses, the 2A peptides allow to link several genes by the consensus motif (2A, Asp-Val/Ile-Glut-X-Asn-Pro-Gly; 2B, Pro) in a single open reading frame (ORF). During translation separate proteins are generated via a process referred to as ribosomal "skipping" [17]. Further marker or functional genes can be included by additional 2A peptides. However, avoid using repetitive sequences in the vector to prevent unwanted recombination events (e.g., employ different 2A peptides like T2A, P2A, F2A, or use alternative codons). Be aware that the size of the insert must not exceed 8 kb, and that expression is reduced with increasing transgene size. DNA preparation for transfection can be performed using a conventional kit (e.g., Qiagen, #12162).

3. Be aware that MLV-eco envelope produced by Plat-E cells is unstable. Half-life of viral particles at 37 °C is about 5–8 h. For short-term storage virus supernatant is best kept on ice, long-term storage requires freezing at −80 °C. Avoid multiple freezing-thawing steps as this dramatically reduces the titer. MLV-eco is not suited for enrichment by ultracentrifugation but might be concentrated with protein filters. Still, optimization of transfection conditions is more likely to yield high-titer virus supernatants than subsequent enrichment steps. We routinely perform large-scale preparation of supernatants, freeze aliquots at −80 °C, and test them on a TCR-deficient T cell line (e.g., 58αβ-cells [18]). These cells express CD3ε when transduced with TCR genes—a convenient surrogate marker in case V-region-specific antibodies are not available. A transduction rate of at least 30–60 % in 58αβ-cells should be achieved with a high-titer supernatant.

4. Although SCA1 is expressed on HSC it is not an exclusive stem cell marker and other bone marrow progenitor cells are similarly SCA1-positive. As to date there is no single cell surface molecule defining HSC, sorting of SCA1-positive cells is one of several options to enrich these cells from total marrow. However, SCA1 is not expressed by all mouse strains. It is found in C57BL/6, but to isolate bone marrow stem cells from BALB/c or BALB/c-derived strains use alternative methods such as positive selection of c-KIT or depletion of lineage marker-positive cells.

## Acknowledgements

This work was supported by DFG grants TR36 and SFB650 (SF) and Hertie Stiftung (SF).

### References

1. Gordon JW, Ruddle FH (1981) Integration and stable germ line transmission of genes injected into mouse pronuclei. Science 214(4526):1244–1246
2. Costantini F, Lacy E (1981) Introduction of a rabbit beta-globin gene into the mouse germ line. Nature 294(5836):92–94
3. Thomas KR, Capecchi MR (1987) Site-directed mutagenesis by gene targeting in mouse embryo-derived stem cells. Cell 51(3): 503–512
4. Kisielow P, Bluthmann H, Staerz UD, Steinmetz M, von Boehmer H (1988) Tolerance in T-cell-receptor transgenic mice involves deletion of nonmature CD4+8+ thymocytes. Nature 333(6175):742–746
5. Joyner A, Keller G, Phillips RA, Bernstein A (1983) Retrovirus transfer of a bacterial gene into mouse haematopoietic progenitor cells. Nature 305(5934):556–558
6. Williams DA, Lemischka IR, Nathan DG, Mulligan RC (1984) Introduction of new genetic material into pluripotent haematopoietic stem cells of the mouse. Nature 310(5977): 476–480
7. Keller G, Paige C, Gilboa E, Wagner EF (1985) Expression of a foreign gene in myeloid and lymphoid cells derived from multipotent haematopoietic precursors. Nature 318(6042):149–154
8. Kang J, Wither J, Hozumi N (1990) Long-term expression of a T-cell receptor beta-chain gene in mice reconstituted with retrovirus-infected hematopoietic stem cells. Proc Natl Acad Sci U S A 87(24):9803–9807
9. Holst J et al (2006) Generation of T-cell receptor retrogenic mice. Nat Protoc 1(1):406–417
10. Holst J, Vignali KM, Burton AR, Vignali DA (2006) Rapid analysis of T-cell selection in vivo using T cell-receptor retrogenic mice. Nat Methods 3(3):191–197
11. Bettini ML, Bettini M, Vignali DA (2012) T-cell receptor retrogenic mice: a rapid, flexible alternative to T-cell receptor transgenic mice. Immunology 136(3):265–272
12. Morita S, Kojima T, Kitamura T (2000) Plat-E: an efficient and stable system for transient packaging of retroviruses. Gene Ther 7(12):1063–1066
13. Baum C, Hegewisch-Becker S, Eckert HG, Stocking C, Ostertag W (1995) Novel retroviral vectors for efficient expression of the multidrug resistance (mdr-1) gene in early hematopoietic cells. J Virol 69(12): 7541–7547
14. Engels B et al (2003) Retroviral vectors for high-level transgene expression in T lymphocytes. Hum Gene Ther 14(12):1155–1168
15. Szymczak AL, Vignali DA (2005) Development of 2A peptide-based strategies in the design of multicistronic vectors. Expert Opin Biol Ther 5(5):627–638
16. Leisegang M et al (2008) Enhanced functionality of T cell receptor-redirected T cells is defined by the transgene cassette. J Mol Med 86(5):573–583
17. Donnelly ML et al (2001) Analysis of the aphthovirus 2A/2B polyprotein 'cleavage' mechanism indicates not a proteolytic reaction, but a novel translational effect: a putative ribosomal 'skip'. J Gen Virol 82(Pt 5):1013–1025
18. Letourneur F, Malissen B (1989) Derivation of a T cell hybridoma variant deprived of functional T cell receptor alpha and beta chain transcripts reveals a nonfunctional alpha-mRNA of BW5147 origin. Eur J Immunol 19(12): 2269–2274

# Chapter 13

# Mouse Models of Allergic Airway Disease

Helen Meyer-Martin, Sebastian Reuter, and Christian Taube

## Abstract

In the last decades there has been a substantial increase in the prevalence of allergic diseases such as asthma. Hence there is a basic necessity to investigate disease mechanisms of allergic disorders and to trace novel treatment approaches. Indeed, allergic asthma is a disorder which is characterized by airway inflammation, airway obstruction, and hyperresponsiveness. Several of these features can be studied in models of allergic airway disease. In this chapter different mouse models of allergic diseases are described. These include frequently models of allergic airway disease utilizing sensitization and challenge towards ovalbumin. Furthermore a model using the human-relevant allergen-specific house dust mite is described. In addition, information about DC-induced models and analysis of in vitro-generated T cell following transfer into recipients are described as well as analysis of a humanized mouse model is provided.

**Key words** Allergic airway disease, Asthma, Mouse models, T cells, Dendritic cells, Humanized mice

## 1 Introduction

The prevalence of asthma has steadily increased over the last decades. Asthma is now the most prevalent chronic disease in childhood in developed countries; approximately 300 million people suffer from this disease worldwide. The Global Initiative of Asthma defines asthma as a chronic inflammatory disorder of the airways. Chronic pulmonary inflammation is associated with airway hyperresponsiveness, which leads to the classical symptoms of asthma: recurrent episodes of wheezing, breathlessness, chest tightness, and coughing (http://www.ginasthma.com). The most common clinical phenotype is allergic asthma. In childhood, more than 90 % of patients with severe asthma are allergic; among asthmatic adults, 60 % are sensitized to common aeroallergens. In allergic asthma, inflammation and airway obstruction are triggered by allergen exposure in atopic individuals. The pathophysiology underlying the disease is rather complex, but development of airway inflammation is a pivotal factor in the development of the disease.

The inflammatory processes underlying the development of allergic airway disease have been investigated in humans and also in

Ari Waisman and Burkhard Becher (eds.), *T-Helper Cells: Methods and Protocols*, Methods in Molecular Biology, vol. 1193,
DOI 10.1007/978-1-4939-1212-4_13, © Springer Science+Business Media New York 2014

animal models of the disease. Indeed, animal models of allergic airway disease have assisted us greatly in gaining a better understanding of the pathophysiological processes underlying asthma development. It is obvious that no single animal model is suited to model all aspects of a disease as complex as human asthma. However, murine models have furthered our understanding of the different cell types and mediators involved in asthma development. Experimental findings support an important role of Th2 cells and Th2 cytokines (IL-4, IL-5, and IL-13) in the development of allergen-induced inflammation and airway hyperresponsiveness (AHR).

Indeed, it is possible to induce several features of asthma in a mouse model, e.g., airway inflammation, airway hyperresponsiveness, and mucus production. These models also allow the investigation of the underlying immunological mechanisms for the development of asthma. Furthermore, it is also possible to assess novel treatment approaches. There is always a huge discussion about the use of these animal models with regard to our understanding of asthma. And certainly these models do not reflect asthma, because it is a very heterogeneous disease, which cannot be reflected in one simple model. However, these models are helpful and necessary to help to understand how cell-to-cell interactions and certain mechanisms occur in a living organism. In this chapter we have collected several methods to induce allergic airway inflammation in mice. This is for sure not a complete collection of all available protocols but offers an overview of models of acute airway inflammation, models for sensitization via the airways, models following transfer of in vitro-polarized T cells, as well as a humanized mouse model of allergic airway disease.

## 2 Acute Model of Allergic Airway Disease

Different murine models of acute asthma inflammation exist and facilitate the investigation of underlying disease mechanisms or therapeutical approaches. One often used model depends on systemic sensitization of naïve mice with a protein, e.g., ovalbumin (OVA), in combination with an adjuvant, for example aluminium hydroxide. These sensitized mice are then subsequently exposed to inhaled protein and develop airway inflammation, AHR, and mucous cell metaplasia.

### 2.1 Materials

| | |
|---|---|
| 1. Animals: | Often this model is performed in C57BL/6 or BALB/c mice, mainly at the age of 8–12 weeks |
| 2. Consumables: | 1 ml Albumin, chicken egg (ovalbumin), grade VI<br>Aluminium hydroxide (e.g., Imject®Alum)<br>0.22 μm filters for sterile filtration |

(continued)

| 3. Buffer and solutions: | |
|---|---|
| Phosphate-buffered saline (PBS): | DPBS 1× |
| OVA stock solution: | 10 mg/ml<br>Use 1× PBS to produce OVA stock solution<br>OVA stock solution should be produced under sterile conditions and afterwards sterile filtrated with 0.22 μm filters |
| OVA/Alum: | 40 μl OVA stock solution<br>960 μl 1× PBS<br>1 ml aluminium hydroxide solution<br>To ensure an optimal homogeneity, solution should be kept warm (37 °C) after production until injection of animals<br>Inject 100 μl per mouse intraperitoneally (i.p.) |

## 2.2 Methods

### 2.2.1 Sensitization Phase

Sensitization is performed on days 0 and 14. Usually, one group is used as a control group which is non-sensitized (injected with PBS) but challenged with the protein (e.g., PBS i.p./OVA challenge). Other mice are sensitized and challenged (e.g., OVA/Alum i.p./OVA challenge).

Inject 100 μl OVA/Alum intraperitoneally on days 0 and 14.

### 2.2.2 Challenge Phase

Challenge is performed on days 28, 29, and 30, and experiments are carried out on day 32. Challenge the animals daily by nebulization with a 1 % OVA solution for 20 min on 3 consecutive days starting 14 days following the second i.p. application. Place animals into a nebulization chamber which is connected to the nebulization device (e.g., ultrasonic nebulizer). Add OVA solution to the medication cup. Inhaled exposure to OVA should be for 20 min.

48 h following last challenge the animals are ready for the analysis.

# 3 Models for Sensitization via Inhalation

The above-described model of allergic airway disease is dependent on systemic sensitization towards a protein and then development of a response in the airways following inhaled exposure. However, the exact route of how sensitization towards a harmless antigen occurs in humans is still under investigation. Epidemiological studies imply that infections of the airways can contribute to the development of an allergic disease of the airway. Viral or bacterial infections, but also bacterial and viral components, can activate the immune system via their pathogen-associated pattern (PAMPS) receptors. Indeed, several studies in the murine model confirm that exposure to a harmless antigen in combination with a PAMP results in an adaptive immune response against the harmless antigen, which leads to sensitization of the organism against this protein.

The following presents two models in which allergic airway disease is induced following an initial inhaled exposure to the allergen and then subsequent repeated reexposures to induce allergic airway disease. Exemplarily one protocol is described for the model antigen OVA. In this model an additional exposure to a viral or a bacterial component (e.g., TLR-4 ligand) is necessary. An additional protocol involves the human-relevant allergen house dust mite (HDM). Interestingly, no additional exposure to a PAMP is necessary as HDM alone leads to an activation of TLR-4 which provides the necessary signal to initialize an immune response [1].

## 3.1 OVA-Specific Sensitization via Inhalation

This protocol is adapted from Nigo et al. [2].

### 3.1.1 Materials

| 1. Animals: | No specific requirement |
|---|---|
| 2. Buffer and solutions: | |
| PBS: | DPBS 1× |
| OVA/LPS: | 1 μg LPS in 25 μl PBS + 10 μg endotoxin-free OVA (in 25 μl PBS per animal) |
| OVA/PBS: | For sensitization: 10 μg endotoxin-free OVA + 50 μl PBS<br>For challenge: 25 μg endotoxin-free OVA + 50 μl PBS |
| Anesthetic: | Ketamine/Rompun; 52.6 vol.% Ketamine Ratiopharm, 21 vol.% Rompun (2 %); 26.3 vol.% PBS |

### 3.1.2 Methods

#### Sensitization Phase

Sensitization is performed on days 1, 2, and 3. Usually, one group is used as a control group which is non-sensitized (exposed to PBS) but challenged with the protein (PBS intranasally (i.n.) during sensitization and OVA/PBS during challenge). Furthermore one group is exposed to OVA alone (OVA/PBS during sensitization and OVA/PBS during challenge), whereas the other group is exposed to OVA in combination with TLR ligand (OVA/LPS during sensitization and OVA/PBS during challenge).

| Preparation: | Prepare the required amount of PBS, OVA/PBS, and OVA/LPS under sterile conditions daily fresh |
|---|---|
| Procedure: | Anesthetize animals. Inject 50 μl/20 g bodyweight i.p.<br>Apply 50 μl of the appropriate solution i.n.<br>Repeat these steps for the following 2 days; change nostril every day<br>If the animal is very small you can apply 25 μl in each nostril every day instead |

#### Challenge Phase

Challenge is performed on days 14, 15, 18, and 19; experiments are performed on day 21.

| Preparation: | Prepare the required amount of OVA/PBS under sterile conditions daily fresh |
|---|---|
| Procedure: | Anesthetize animals<br>Inject 50 μl/20 g bodyweight i.p.<br>Apply 50 μl of the OVA/PBS solution i.n.<br>Repeat these steps on days 15, 18, and 19<br>Experiments can be performed on day 21 |

### 3.2 HDM-Specific Sensitization via Inhalation

This model is adapted from Willart et al. [3].

#### 3.2.1 Materials

| 1. Animals: | No specific requirement |
|---|---|
| 2. Buffer and solutions: | |
| PBS: | DPBS 1× |
| HDM/PBS: | Sensitization:<br>1 μg HDM (e.g., *Dermatophagoides pteronyssinus* extracts) in 80 μl PBS per mouse<br>Challenge:<br>10 μg HDM (e.g., *Dermatophagoides pteronyssinus* extracts) in 80 μl PBS per mouse |
| Anesthetic: | Isoflurane |

#### 3.2.2 Methods

Sensitization Phase

Sensitization is performed on day 1. As groups use at least unsensitized (PBS i.n. during sensitization and HDM/PBS during challenge) and HDM-sensitized (HDM/PBS during sensitization and HDM/PBS during challenge) animals.

| Preparation: | Prepare the required amount of PBS and HDM/PBS under sterile conditions |
|---|---|
| Procedure: | Anesthetize animals with isoflurane<br>Apply 80 μl of the appropriate solution i.n.<br>If the animal is very small you can apply 40 μl in each nostril every day |

Challenge Phase

Challenge is performed on days 7–11; experiment is performed on day 14.

| Preparation: | Prepare the required amount of HDM/PBS under sterile conditions daily fresh |
|---|---|
| Procedure: | Anesthetize animals with isoflurane<br>Apply 80 μl of the HDM/PBS solution i.n.<br>Repeat these steps on days 8–11<br>Experiment can be performed on day 14 |

## 4 T Cell-Depending Model of an Allergic Airway Disease

In recent years it became clear that besides the well-described Th2-mediated inflammation also other T cell populations can contribute to inflammatory asthmatic phenotypes. Besides Th2 also Th9 cells have been shown to induce an allergic airway inflammation which is also characterized by increased numbers of eosinophils in the airways. In contrast, allergen-specific Th1 as well as Th17 cells induce a neutrophilic inflammation in the airways following allergen exposure. To analyze the specific role of the different polarized T cell populations it is possible to use mice carrying the MHC class II-restricted rearranged T cell receptor transgene, which reacts to ovalbumin (OVA) peptide antigen. These T cells can be isolated, polarized in vitro, and then transferred into immune-incompetent hosts. These recipients are then exposed to repeated inhaled allergen exposure (e.g., for 6 subsequent days). With this model analysis of polarized T cells in vivo is possible and the effect of certain interventions (e.g., pharmacological, transfer of other cell populations) can be assessed.

### *4.1 Materials*

| | |
|---|---|
| 1. Animals: | OVA transgenic OTII mice as T cell donors<br>Rag—deficient mice (lacking T and B cells) (B6/J) as recipients<br>Or OVA transgenic Balb/c DO11.10 mice as T cell donors<br>Rag—deficient mice (lacking T and B cells) (Balb/c) as recipients |
| 2. Equipment: | MACS magnet [MACS Miltenyi Biotec] |
| 3. Consumables: | MACS separation column 25 LS [MACS Miltenyi Biotec]<br>Tube: pp-tubes, sterile, 50 ml, cell strainer 70 μm nylon, cell strainer 40 μm nylon<br>24-well cell culture plate |
| 4. Buffer and solutions: | |
| BSA: | Albumin from bovine serum |
| PBS: | DPBS 1× |
| IMDM: | Iscove's Modified Dulbecco's Medium<br>Tween 20 |
| Gey's solution: | 10 mM $KHCO_3$, 155 mM $NH_4Cl$, 100 μM ethylenediaminetetraacetic acid (EDTA) |
| GM buffer: | 0.5 % BSA; 0.001 % sodium acid, 5 mM EDTA in 1× PBS |
| Test medium 5 (TM5): | IMDM including 5 % (v/v) FCS, 4 mM L-glutamine solution, 1 mM sodium pyruvate |
| Th2 cytokine mix: | 10,000 U/ml murine (mr) IL-4, 200 μg/ml XMG 8a-IFN-γ, 1,000 U/ml mr-IL6 in TM5 |
| Th2 feeding medium: | TM5 including 200 U/ml mr IL-4, 100 U/ml human (h) IL-2 (proleucine), 100 U/ml mr IL-6 |

(continued)

| | |
|---|---|
| Thl cytokine mix: | TM5 including 3,000 U/ml mr-IL-12, 10 μg/ml α-IL4, 1,000 U/ml proleucine (hIL-2) |
| Thl feeding medium: | TM5 including 100 U/ml proleucine |
| Column wash medias: | PBS/BSA:<br>0.5 % BSA in PBS |
| PBS/FCS: | 10 % FCS in PBS |
| Working medium (WM): | DMEM<br>+ 2 % (v/v) FCS |
| Antibodies/beads: | αCD25 (PC61 bio) 0.5 μg/ml<br>αCD4 (H129.19 bio) 0.5 μg/ml<br>SA-beads: Streptavidin micro beads, MACS Miltenyi Biotec |

## 4.2 Methods

### 4.2.1 Isolation of Spleen Cells

All preparation steps are performed under sterile conditions

1. Preparation
   - Disinfect set of instrument; carry out all products at room temperature.
   - Prepare for each expected spleen a petri dish filled with 5 ml WM, and place the cell strainer into the dish.
2. Taxidermy
   - Kill the mouse (OTII/DO11.10, respectively) by cervical dislocation.
   - Disinfect the skin and open the abdomen.
   - Take the spleen out and grind it via a stamp of a 10 ml syringe through the prepared cell strainer (70 μm) into the petri dish.
   - Transfer the suspension into a tube and wash the filter with additional 5 ml WM, to take also the residual cells.
   - To sediment big particles incubate cells for 5 min at 4 °C.
   - Convey supernatant with cells carefully into a new tube.
3. Cell lysis and adjustment
   - Centrifuge at 1,400 rpm (411 ×$g$), 4 °C, for 8 min; if not indicated use this setting also in other steps.
   - Abolish the supernatant and resuspend the pellet in 1 ml Gey's lysis for 1 min.
   - Stop the reaction with 5 ml MEM and transfer suspension through a 70 μm filter into a new tube.
   - Centrifuge and wash two times with WM.
   - Count cells and adjust up to $1 \times 10^8$ cells/ml in GM buffer.

### 4.2.2 CD4 Isolation

4. Preparation
   - Prepare MACS separation columns (flush column: fill it unto top with PBS/Tween, wait until it passes through; repeat

this step with PBS, ethanol, and at last 5 ml PBS/BSA); you need three columns per $5 \times 10^8$ cells.

- Attach the separation column to the MACS magnet; place a 15 ml reaction tube under each column.

5. Procedure

- Centrifuge adjusted cell suspension at 1,700 rpm ($600 \times g$), 4 °C, for 6 min; use this setting as from now.
- Break pellet and adjust cells again to $1 \times 10^8$ cells/ml in GM buffer.
- Add 0.5 μg αCD25 bio/$1 \times 10^8$ cells and incubate at 4 °C for 20 min.
- Meanwhile prepare plates for cell culture.
- Coat a 24-well cell culture plate with α-CD3 (concentration 3 μg/ml) in 500 μl PBS/well for a minimum 30 min at 37 °C.
- Continue with isolation, wash cells, add 5 ml GM buffer, centrifuge suspension, discard supernatant, and repeat this step twice.
- Break pellet and add the volume of GM buffer to receive $1 \times 10^8$ cells/ml.
- Add SA beads at the ratio 1/20 to the cell suspension and incubate for 20 min at 4 °C.
- Transfer suspension through a 40 μm filter into a new tube.
- Wash the tube with GM buffer again and transfer the flush; the end volume should be 5 ml.
- Pipet the suspension in 1 ml steps through the separation column, which is attached to the MACS magnet.
- Irrigate tube with $2 \times 3$ ml GM buffer and transfer it to the separation column too.
- Collect the flow through in the already prepared 15 ml reaction tube.
- For the next steps use only the flow through (CD25-negative population) collected in the 15 ml reaction tube. The CD25-positive cells which are associated to the beads will remain in the column adhered by the magnetic field.
- Centrifuge, count cells, and adjust to $1 \times 10^8$ cell/ml in GM buffer.
- Incubate suspension with 0.5 μg αCD4 bio/ml for 15 min at 4 °C.
- Meanwhile continue the preparation of the culture plate.

- Wash the coated 24-well cell culture plate three times by flushing each well with PBS (1 ml), refill the wells with 500 μl of α-CD28/PBS solution (concentration 10 μg/ml), and incubate for at least 30 min at 37 °C.
- Continue with CD4 isolation: Add 5 ml GM buffer, centrifuge suspension, discard supernatant, and repeat this step twice.
- Break the pellet and add the volume to adjust cells to $1 \times 10^8$ cells/ml.
- Add SA beads (1/40) and incubate for 15 min at 4 °C.
- Adjust to a final volume of 5 ml with GM buffer.
- Pipet the suspension in 1 ml steps through the second separation column.
- Wash tube again two times with 3 ml GM buffer und transfer it also to the column.
- Discard the 15 ml tube with the flow through.
- Remove the separation column from the MACS magnet and place it on a new tube.
- Elute cells with 5 ml GM from the column (eluate I).
- To improve purity, use eluate I and repeat the last five steps use the third separation column, and elute again (eluate II).
- Centrifuge eluate II, wash with TM5, count, and adjust to $1 \times 10^7$ cells/ml TM5.

6. Purity check
   - Purity should be checked via FACS; use antibodies against CD4/CD8/CD3 and CD25. Cells should be CD4/CD3 positive and CD8/CD25 negative.

*4.2.3 Th2/Th1 Differentiation*

7. Procedure
   - Wash the already prepared cell culture plate three times by flushing each well with 1 ml PBS.
   - Fill well with 800 μl TM5, 100 μl appropriate cytokine mix (Th1/Th2), and 100 μl cell suspension (final $1 \times 10^6$ cells/well).
   - To support the cell/coat interaction, centrifuge plate for 2 min at 400 rpm ($34 \times g$) at 4 °C. Incubate the plates for 3 days at 37 °C in an incubator (5 % $CO_2$).
   - Transfer and split cells into new uncoated wells. Resuspend accurately to dissolve the cells from the coat.
   - Feed cells with 500 μl of the appropriate Th1/Th2 medium.
   - Repeat the incubation until day 6.

8. Purity check
   - Intracellular FACS staining should be performed; surface antibodies against CD3/CD4 and intracellular antibodies against IL-5, IL-13, and IFN-γ are recommended.
     - Th1 population: CD3/CD4 positive; IFN-γ positive/IL-5, IL-13 negative.
     - Th2 population: CD3/CD4 positive; IL-5, IL-13 positive/IFN-γ negative.
   - Cytokine profile can also be checked in the supernatants via ELISA.

*4.2.4 Application and Asthma Model*

9. Application
   - Transfer Th1 and Th2 cells, respectively, into a 50 ml tube.
   - Add 10 ml PBS and wash cells twice at 1,200 rpm ($300 \times g$) for 8 min and 4 °C.
   - Determine cell count and adjust cells to $2 \times 10^7$/ml PBS.
   - Inject 100 μl of the cell suspension ($2 \times 10^6$ cells) intravenously into the tail vein of T cell/B cell-deficient $Rag^{-/-}$ animals.
10. Treatment protocol
   - Challenge the animals daily by nebulization with a 1 % OVA solution for 20 min on 6 consecutive days starting 24 h following i.v. application. Place animals into a nebulization chamber which is connected to the nebulization device (e.g., OMRON ultrasonic nebulizer NE-U17). Add 30 ml OVA solution to the medication cup. Set timer to 20 min and airflow volume and nebulization volume to 6.
   - 24 h following last challenge the animals are ready for the analysis.

## 5 DC-Depending Model of an Allergic Airway Disease

Dendritic cells (DCs) play an essential role for the induction of adaptive immune responses. The following protocol is adapted from Idzko et al. [4] and can be used to analyze DC-mediated effects in the airway disease. For this DCs are derived from culturing bone marrow cells. These DCs are then in vitro loaded with the antigen. These antigen-loaded DCs are installed into the lungs of animals. Several days following the DCs application animals are exposed to inhaled antigen, which then leads to the development of allergic airway disease. By generating DCs from gene-deficient animals or pretreatment of bone marrow-derived dendritic cells (BMDC) in vitro with pharmaceuticals this approach can be utilized to assess the role of different pathways in DCs for the development of allergic airway disease.

## 5.1 Materials

| | |
|---|---|
| 1. Animals: | Animals with a congenic background should be chosen as donors and recipients to avoid alloreactions |
| 2. Equipment: | Vessel scissors—one blade probe pointed scissor<br>Delicate scissors—straight<br>Dissecting and Strabismus scissors—straight<br>Tweezers—fine<br>Tweezers—rough |
| 3. Consumables: | Cell strainer—sterile (0.7 μm)<br>Syringe—sterile (5–10 ml)<br>Cannula (0.7 × 30 mm)<br>Three petri dishes |
| 4. Buffer and solutions: | |
| Working medium (WM): | DMEM including 2 % (v/v) FCS, 1 % penicillin-streptomycin (P/S stock solution 10,000 U/ml penicillin/10 mg/ml streptomycin) |
| Test medium (TM): | IMDM including 10 % (v/v) FCS, 1 % L-glutamine solution (stock: 200 mM), 50 μM mercaptoethanol, 1 % P/S solution |
| Gey's solution: | 10 mM potassium hydrogen carbonate ($KHCO_3$)<br>155 mM ammonium chloride ($NH_4Cl$)<br>100 μM ethylenediaminetetraacetic acid $C_{10}H_{14}N_2O_5Na_2 \times 2H_2O$ in aqua dest., pH 7.5 |
| Anesthetic: | Ketamine/Rompun; 52.6 vol.% Ketamine Ratiopharm, 21 vol.% Rompun (2 %); 26.3 vol.% PBS |
| OVA stock: | 10 mg OVA/ml PBS sterile filtered |
| OVA challenge-solution: | 1 % w/v OVA solution. 0.3 g OVA diluted in 30 ml PBS |
| GM-CSF: | Supernatant of GM-CSF-transfected X63.Ag8-653 cell line |

## 5.2 Methods

All preparation steps are performed under sterile condition.

### 5.2.1 Preparation of Bone Marrow Cells

1. Preparation
   - Prepare three petri dishes; fill petri dish I with EtOH (70 %), and fill petri dish II and III each with WM.
2. Taxidermy
   - Crucify mice by cervical dislocation.
   - Wet the animal with alcohol (70 %).
   - Remove the skin around the legs.
   - Take a foot and pull the leg firmly towards head until it dislocates.
   - Remove the foot by twisting it carefully; if necessary cut tendon with delicate scissors.

- Remove flesh from the bones and dislocate carefully femur and tibia.
- Sterilize bones by dipping them into petri dish I.
- Collect all bones in petri dish II until all animals are prepared.
- Remove the remaining flesh by rubbing them between an EtOH-soaked tissue.
- Take single bone cut off carefully from upper and lower joint head.
- Fill syringe with WM and flush via the cannula the bone marrow into the petri dish III.
- Repeat the last three steps with all bones.
- Resuspend bone marrow cells with the syringe at least five times.
- Transfer via pipette cells over a cell strainer into a 50 ml reaction tube.
- Wash dish with additionally 10 ml WM and transfer the solution also over the strainer into the tube.
- Centrifuge cells at 1,200 rpm ($242 \times g$) for 8–10 min at 4 °C.
- Discard the supernatant and break pellet.

3. Cell lysis and adjustment
   - Add Gey's solution (1 ml per BM of 1–2 mice) for 1 min to lyse red blood cells.
   - To stop the lysis add at least 10 ml WM.
   - Centrifuge cells at 1,200 rpm ($242 \times g$) for 8–10 min at 4 °C.
   - Discard the supernatant and break pellet; the pellet should be now almost white.
   - Repeat the washing steps twice.
   - After the final wash add 10 ml WM and analyze the cell count.
   - Adjust cells to $2 \times 10^6$ cells per ml TM.

#### 5.2.2 BMDC Culture

4. Procedure
   - For the cell culture $2 \times 10^6$ cells per petri dish are used in a total volume of 10 ml TM supplemented with 5 % GM-CSF.
   - Pipette 1 ml of the adjusted cells per petri dish, and add 8.5 ml TM and 0.5 ml GM-CSF.
   - Incubate dishes at 37 °C and 5 % $CO_2$ in an incubator.

- Cells should be supplied with fresh medium on days 3 and 6; on day 8 90 % of the cells should be differentiated into DC.
- Cultures should be checked daily for cell density and size.
- Day 3: Add 10 ml TM (37 °C)+5 % GM-CSF to each petri dish.
- Day 6: Take 10 ml cell suspension from each petri dish and collect them in a 50 ml reaction tube. Centrifuge tubes at (242 ×*g* for 10 min. Discard supernatants, and break the pellet and the same volume of TM (37 °C)+5 % GM-CSF which was before discarded.
- Add 10 ml of the fresh cell suspension to each petri dish.
- Day 8: BMDC culture is ready, and purity should be checked by FACS.

5. Purity check
   - To analyze the purity of your culture perform a FACS staining with antibodies against CD11c and MHCII.
   - Cells should be positive for both markers.
   - You can check marker expression also following OVA loading (**step 6**); expression of MHCII should be slightly upregulated in OVA-treated DC in comparison to untreated DC.

### 5.2.3 BMDC Antigen Loading and Application

6. BMDC antigen loading
   - Add OVA solution to the cell culture (200 μg/ml).
   - Incubate cells overnight.
   - Collect all cells from the same treatment group.
   - Wash cells twice with PBS; centrifuge cells at 1,200 rpm (242 ×*g*) for 8–10 min at 4 °C.
   - Discard supernatant and add 10 ml PBS.
   - Adjust cells to $1.25 \times 10^7$ cells/ml PBS.
7. Application and treatment protocol
   - Anesthetize animals.
   - Inject 50 μl/20 g bodyweight i.p.
   - Apply 40 μl of the adjusted DC solution in the nostril of the animals. Wait until breathing pattern returns to normal and repeat the procedure with the other nostril so that overall $1 \times 10^6$ DCs are installed into each animal.
   - As a negative group administer also naïve untreated DC.
   - Challenge the animals daily by nebulization with a 1 % OVA solution for 20 min on 3 consecutive days starting on day 10. Place animals into a nebulization chamber which is

connected to the nebulization device (e.g., ultrasonic nebulizer). Add 30 ml OVA solution to the medication cup. Set timer to 20 min and airflow volume and nebulization volume to 6.

- 48 h following the last challenge animals can be analyzed.

## 6 A Humanized Mouse Model of Allergic Airway Disease: Purification of Human Peripheral Blood Mononuclear Cells (PBMCs) from Allergic Donors and Transfer into Immunodeficient Mice

The following model enables the investigation of allergic disease mediated from human cells in immunodeficient mice. It is a more translational model that can be used for investigation of human cell interactions in vivo and the influence of medical substances on the development of allergic airway disease. The occurring inflammation in the model depends on human T cells that should be isolated from the blood of patients with stable allergic asthma (in accordance with the Global Initiative for Asthma guidelines, http://www.ginaasthma.com). In the present situation cells were isolated from patients with birch allergy [5, 6]. For exposure in the animals birch allergen was used. However, other models utilized cells from patients sensitized to house dust mite [7, 8].

### 6.1 Materials

| | |
|---|---|
| 1. Animals: | Mouse strain: NOD-Scid γc (Nod.Cg-Prkdc scid Il2rg tm 1 Wjl/SzJ), adult mice (8–12 weeks old) |
| 2. Consumables: | Sterile 50 ml tubes |
| 3. Buffer and solutions | |
| Anticlotting buffer: | For dilution of buffy coats or whole-blood samples use 1× PBS, 0.4 % Liquemin® (Heparin-Natrium-2500, 2 mM EDTA) |
| Wash buffer: | 1× PBS, 1 mM EDTA |
| Ficoll: | 1.077 for Ficoll density centrifugation |
| | Human IL-4 |
| | Lyophilized allergen |
| Anesthetic: | Isoflurane |

### 6.2 Methods

Purification of PBMCs from human blood of asthmatic individuals with sensitization against birch (high specific IgE levels, CAP 4-6) by Ficoll high-density centrifugation.

1. Procedure
   - Collect blood in heparinized syringes.
   - Dilute 12 ml heparinized blood in 10 ml PBS, 0.4 Vol% Liquemin®, and 2 mM EDTA; use 50 ml Falcon tubes.

- Underlay suspension with 10 ml Ficoll.
- Be careful and avoid mixing Ficoll and blood suspension.
- Centrifuge tubes: Centrifuge at room temperature, 800 × *g*, for 20 min without brake.
- After centrifugation transfer cells from the cloudy layer below the upper plasma phase in a fresh 50 ml Falcon tube with PBS/EDTA and wash cells in 50 ml PBS/EDTA till supernatant is clear (at least three times, centrifugation at 4 °C, 411 × *g*, for 8 min).
- Attention with decanting supernatant after the first washing step: Pellet is not really fixed on the bottom of the tube.
- For injection resuspend $5 \times 10^6$ PBMCs with recombinant human IL-4 (10 ng) and birch allergen (20 μg) and inject them intraperitoneally into the mice (total injection volume 200–300 μl).
- 7 days later boost mice intraperitoneally by injection of 10 ng IL-4 and 20 μg birch allergen diluted in 20 μl PBS.
- On days 20–22 treat the mice once every day by intranasal application of 20 μg birch allergen diluted in 20 μl PBS; mice should be anesthetized for challenge by inhalation of isoflurane.
- Mice can be analyzed for 48 h after the last intranasal challenge.

## References


1. Hammad H, Chieppa M, Perros F, Willart MA, Germain RN, Lambrecht BN (2009) House dust mite allergen induces asthma via Toll-like receptor 4 triggering of airway structural cells. Nat Med 15:410
2. Nigo YI, Yamashita M, Hirahara K, Shinnakasu R, Inami M, Kimura M, Hasegawa A, Kohno Y, Nakayama T (2006) Regulation of allergic airway inflammation through Toll-like receptor 4-mediated modification of mast cell function. Proc Natl Acad Sci U S A 103:2286
3. Willart MA, Deswarte K, Pouliot P, Braun H, Beyaert R, Lambrecht BN, Hammad H (2012) Interleukin-1 alpha controls allergic sensitization to inhaled house dust mite via the epithelial release of GM-CSF and IL-33. J Exp Med 209:1505
4. Idzko M, Hammad H, van Nimwegen M, Kool M, Vos N, Hoogsteden HC, Lambrecht BN (2007) Inhaled iloprost suppresses the cardinal features of asthma via inhibition of airway dendritic cell function. J Clin Invest 117:464
5. Bellinghausen I, Reuter S, Martin H, Maxeiner J, Luxemburger U, Tureci O, Grabbe S, Taube C, Saloga J (2012) Enhanced production of CCL18 by tolerogenic dendritic cells is associated with inhibition of allergic airway reactivity. J Allergy Clin Immunol 130:1384
6. Martin H, Reuter S, Dehzad N, Heinz A, Bellinghausen I, Saloga J, Haasler I, Korn S, Jonuleit H, Buhl R, Becker C, Taube C (2012) CD4-mediated regulatory T-cell activation inhibits the development of disease in a humanized mouse model of allergic airway disease. J Allergy Clin Immunol 129(521):528
7. Duez C, Kips J, Pestel J, Tournoy K, Tonnel AB, Pauwels R (2000) House dust mite-induced airway changes in hu-SCID mice. Am J Respir Crit Care Med 161:200
8. Hammad H, Lambrecht BN, Pochard P, Gosset P, Marquillies P, Tonnel AB, Pestel J (2002) Monocyte-derived dendritic cells induce a house dust mite-specific Th2 allergic inflammation in the lung of humanized SCID mice: involvement of CCR7. J Immunol 169:1524

# Chapter 14

# Induction of Colitis in Mice (T-Cell Transfer Model)


## Benno Weigmann



## Abstract

Animal model of intestinal inflammation is essential for the understanding of the pathomechanisms of inflammatory bowel diseases like Crohn's disease and ulcerative colitis. Typically, naïve T-cells were transferred into immunocompromised mice and develop gut inflammation because of inappropriate downregulation. Here, we describe the isolation, purification, and transfer of $CD4^{+}CD25^{-}$ T-cells into recipients to obtain an experimental colitis model for the analysis of pathogenesis.



**Key words** Inflammatory bowel disease, Experimental colitis model, SCID, RAG, Naïve T-cells, FACS, MACS


## 1 Introduction

Crohn's disease and ulcerative colitis are chronic inflammatory disorders of the intestine [1]. The etiology of IBD still remains unclear, but common understanding is that immunocompetent cells, especially T-cells, contribute to disease initiation and progression. Much of the recent progress in the understanding of mucosal immunity has been achieved by analysis of experimental animal models of intestinal inflammation [2]. Most of these models are based on immune cell transfer or chemical induction. Nevertheless, these models do not fully represent the complexity of human disease; they are valuable tools for understanding the pathophysiological mechanisms. However, it is still incompletely understood whether disease results in a persistent activation of the mucosal immune system. Intestinal immune cell populations and cytokines have been characterized in humans over a long time and studies of animal models emphasized the evidence of immune cell activation or inappropriate downregulation resulting in the induction of mucosal inflammation. T-lymphocytes, in particular $CD4^{+}$ T-cells, play a key role in all immune-regulatory processes in the gastrointestinal tract [3]. Whereas the activation of innate immune cells is a common feature of IBD, different T-cell subsets are present and


Ari Waisman and Burkhard Becher (eds.), *T-Helper Cells: Methods and Protocols*, Methods in Molecular Biology, vol. 1193, DOI 10.1007/978-1-4939-1212-4_14, © Springer Science+Business Media New York 2014

activated, indicating the failure of regulation by Th cells. In inflamed mucosa of Crohn's disease patients a production of IFN-γ, TNF-α, and IL-12p40 has been observed which is consistent with a Th1-related response [4]. An exaggerated Th1-type response has been described as a main feature in the induction of inflammation in most experimental animal models [5]. Because of these observations, together with a more precisely synchronized onset and severity of the disease, the T-cell transfer model has become used over the last years [6]. This well-characterized colitis model induced the disruption of the T-cell homeostasis. Adaptive transfer of naïve T-cells from healthy wild-type mice into syngeneic recipients that lack T and B cells induces a pancolitis at 5–8 weeks following T-cell transfer [7]. Histopathological analysis of the colon obtained from mice with active disease reveals a transmural inflammation, epithelial cell hyperplasia, infiltration of leukocyte crypt abscesses, and epithelial erosions. Due to frequent use, studies described that inflammation can be observed in colon and induction of inflammation is localized also in small bowel, making this model similar to Crohn's disease. Secondary parameters of the inflammation can be observed by varying weight loss and loose stools. The major advantage of the transfer model is that the very early immunological events are associated with the induction of inflammation and the perpetuation of the disease. This model is ideal to study the role of regulatory T-cells playing more suppressive or limiting function of the onset and the perpetuation of intestinal and colonic inflammation. There exist different models, which differ in the transferred cell population. First, user isolated $CD4^{+}CD45RBhigh$ or $CD4^{+}CD62L^{+}$ naïve T-cells and purified cells with a FACS-Sorter. Later, naïve T-cells marked as $CD4^{+}CD25^{-}$ can be more easily purified with the magnetic bead technique, combined with a high purity. Therefore, we describe here the $CD4^{+}CD25^{-}$ colitis transfer model.

## 2 Materials

### 2.1 Equipment

1. Centrifuge with swinging bucket refrigerated.
2. Platform shaker.
3. Magnet for isolation cells (Miltenyi Biotec).
4. Cell strainer 100 μm (BD).

### 2.2 Animals

1. C57BL/6 wt mice or BALB/c wt mice of either sex are used as donors.
2. Immunodeficient RAG $1^{-/-}$ mice (male) on C57BL/6 background or SCID mice on BALB/c background used for recipients. If you use female or male donor wt mice, then you can use as recipient male mice. If only female recipient mice are available, then only female wt donors should be used.

### 2.3 Reagents

1. MACS buffer: 1× PBS (without $Ca^{2+}$) supplemented with 3 % fetal calf serum and 2 mM EDTA. Prepare all solutions with sterile conditions and store all reagents at 4 °C (unless indicated otherwise).
2. FACS buffer: 1× PBS (without $Ca^{2+}$) supplemented with 2 % fetal calf serum.
3. ACK (ammonium-chloride-potassium) buffer: 0.15 M Ammonium chloride ($NH_4Cl$), 10 mM potassium hydrogen carbonate ($KHCO_3$), and 0.1 mM EDTA, adjust pH with NaOH/HCl to 7.2 $CD4^+CD25^+$ regulatory T-cell isolation kit mouse (MACS).
4. Fluorescence-labelled antibodies for the detection of T-cell surface markers, such as CD4-FITC and CD25-APC. These antibodies are for testing the purity of the isolated cells.
5. Trypan blue solution: Prepare in 1× PBS with 0.4 % (w/v).

## 3 Methods

1. Because of living cells, all steps of the method should be done on ice unless otherwise specified.
2. We enrich $CD4^+$ cells in first step by negative selection with magnetic beads.
3. In the second step $CD4^+CD25^-$ will be enriched by eliminating $CD4^+CD25^+$ T-cells. After the procedure the success of the cell enrichment is analyzed by FACS measuring.

### 3.1 Enrichment of the CD4+ T-Cells

1. Remove spleens and put them into a petri dish with 10 ml MACS buffer.
2. Take two moistened glass slides and take the spleen between the rough ends. Start rubbing until the connective tissue capsule remains. Go further on rubbing with large pieces until a homogeneous cell suspension is remaining.
3. Give now the cell suspension with a pipette over the 100 μm cell strainer and let it pass through into a 15 ml tube.
4. Pellet cells by centrifugation at $400 \times g$ for 10 min at 4 °C.
5. Aspirate and discard the supernatant and resuspend the cells with 2 ml ACK buffer. The buffer lyses the red blood cells by hypotonic effect.
6. Gently disrupt the cell pellet by pipetting for 60 s.
7. Add at once 8 ml MACS buffer and pellet the cells by centrifugation at $400 \times g$ for 10 min at 4 °C.
8. Aspirate and discard the supernatant and resuspend the cell pellet with pipette in 10 ml MACS buffer.

9. Centrifuge the cell suspension at 400 × *g* for 10 min at 4 °C.
10. Aspirate and discard the supernatant.
11. Resuspend the cells in 10 ml MACS buffer and count the cells by Trypan blue staining method. In brief, vortex cell suspension and transfer 10 μl into a 2 ml tube containing 90 μl Trypan blue solution (resulting in a dilution of 1:10). Mix gently the cells and transfer cell suspension to hemocytometer chamber. Count and calculate viable cells by using a cell microscope.
12. Centrifuge the cell suspension at 400 × *g* for 10 min at 4 °C.
13. Aspirate and discard the supernatant.
14. Resuspend the cell pellet in 500 μl MACS buffer. Take a small amount of 10 μl cell suspension in a new 2 ml tube and save them for later FACS analysis on ice.
15. Now use the MACS CD4 CD25 regulatory T-cell isolation kit protocol for further enrichment of $CD4^{+}CD25^{-}$ T-cells. Do all incubation steps on a soft shaking or rocking platform with ice to achieve best binding possibility of the beads. By using this isolation kit the T-cells are untouched by antibodies because of binding the non-$CD4^{+}$ cells and isolating the non-$CD25^{+}$ cells as flow through. Take from the $CD4^{+}$, $CD4^{-}$, $CD25^{+}$, and $CD25^{-}$ fraction a small amount for FACS analysis (*see* **step 14**).
16. Pellet cells by centrifugation at 400 × *g* at 4 °C for 10 min.
17. Aspirate, discard the supernatant, and resuspend the cell pellet in 1 ml PBS. If clumps are visible then pass the cell suspension through a 100 μm cell strainer.
18. Count the cells by Trypan blue staining method (*see* **step 11**).

### 3.2 FACS Analysis of the Isolated Cells

1. Prepare the CD4-FITC and CD25-APC antibodies in an optimal dilution (accordingly to the antibody concentration) with PBS. To do this, add appropriate amount of antibody to a 2 ml tube, add 1 ml PBS, and vortex well.
2. Take the small amounts of different fractions and transfer to 5 ml FACS tubes with 200 μl FACS buffer (*see* Subheading 3.1, **steps 14** and **15**).
3. Add the calculated antibody cocktail for each tube and mix by pipetting several times up and down.
4. Incubate tubes on a rocking platform for 15 min at 4 °C.
5. Wash by filling each tube with 1 ml FACS buffer.
6. Pellet cells by centrifugation tubes at 400 × *g* at 4 °C for 10 min.
7. Aspirate and discard the supernatant.
8. Resuspend the cells in 300 μl FACS buffer and vortex.
9. Start the FACS analysis by adjusting of SSC and FSC parameters. A sample of unstained cells is useful to gate the lymphoid cells and to discriminate dead or debris from measurement.

10. Single-color controls are useful to establish the compensation levels of fluorochrome, especially by using other dyes than FITC and APC dye. Normally, no compensation with the combination of FITC and APC is necessary.
11. Create a single histogram with FACS instrument software with respect to lymphoid cells gated in SSC/FSC dot blot and use a gate for $CD4^{-}FITC^{+}$ cells. Normally approx. 25 % of the analyzed cells should be positive.
12. Make a second single histogram for $CD25\text{-}APC^{+}$ cells, gated on $CD4^{+}$ cells. Normally approx. 50 % of the analyzed cells should be positive.
13. Analyze now all samples taken from cell separation and measure the percentage of CD4 and CD25 for purity. If the percentage of $CD4^{+}CD25^{-}$ cells is high, e.g., >98 %, then cells are pure and can be used for the transfer colitis model. If purity is less, then repeat cell separation until purity is high enough.
14. Count the cell number (*see* Subheading 3.1, **step 11**).

### 3.3 Adoptive Transfer of Purified $CD4^{+}CD25^{-}$ Cells to Immunocompromised Mice

1. Fill the purified $CD4^{+}CD25^{-}$ T-cells with 5 ml 1× PBS buffer and pellet cells by centrifugation at $400 \times g$ at 4 °C for 10 min.
2. Aspirate and discard the supernatant. Resuspend the cells by gently pipetting with 1× PBS and calculate the liquid volume with a final concentration of $2 \times 10^{6}$ cell/ml. The cell suspension should be stored prior to injection always on ice.
3. Take a syringe (with 1 ml volume and Luer Solo connection) with a 26G×1″ needle and draw carefully 0.6 ml of the cell suspension. Hold the mouse on the neck and stretch the animal by pushing gently the abdomen with the fingers. Inject carefully 0.5 ml cell suspension i.p. (intraperitoneally) into the recipient mice. By using a higher angle of the injection needle to the mouse the danger of subcutaneous injection will be reduced.
4. Weight the recipient mice with a balance and record the weight in order to get the starting weight.
5. Monitor the character of the colonic mucosa by using the colonoscopy (Coloview). By this, a precise sight at the mucosa is possible and the beginning of or ongoing inflammation can be observed in a better way.

### 3.4 Evaluation of the Progressing Inflammation and Finalization of the Experiment

1. Normally, the weight of the animals will increase in the first 3 weeks and then, be aware that weight loss will occur in the next 4–6 weeks. These symptoms will be accompanied with diarrhea and a possibly more hunched appearance. Monitor the progression of the disease by taking the weight of the animals twice a week (*see* **Note 1**).

2. Monitor the animals by doing colonoscopy once a week. Score the condition of the mucosa by making the MEICS score, based on five parameters (translucency, granularity, fibrin production, vascularity, and consistence of the stool). The scoring system allows you to give number starting from 0 to 3 for each parameter. At least you get a sum of all parameters and you can clearly distinguish between the states of inflammation in individual animals (*see* **Note 2**).
3. If mice lose more than 15 % of their starting body weight, then animals should be euthanized and the experiment should be finalized. By finalizing, tissue, blood, and organs from animals are prepared to do afterwards analysis.
4. Open the abdomen of the mouse by using surgical scissors and prepare the entire colon. This can be done by cutting the colon below the cecum and around the anus.
5. Lay the entire colon carefully on a paper, clean it from fecal material by squeezing the pellets out, and measure the length without stretching. Signs of inflammation are the shortening of the colon and thickening of the bowel wall.
6. After that, a piece of colon should be excised carefully and should be snap-frozen. From this colonic tissue a cryo-section is manufactured in order to stain histopathological scoring, e.g., H&E staining (hematoxylin and eosin staining) (*see* **Note 3**).
7. Remaining pieces of the colon can be stored for analysis of mRNA in RNA stabilization reagent immediately or for the preparation of mucosal cells in 1× PBS.
8. For the analysis of inflammatory cytokines in serum collecting of blood should be done. Because of the quick agglutination process a prompt action is necessary. By using a syringe (10 ml volume with an 18G × 1″ needle) a punctuation of the heart is done, in order to get access to the heart ventricle. Typically, 1–2 ml blood is collected. After collecting the blood place the tube in an upright position at room temperature and incubate for 30–45 min (no longer than 60 min) to allow clotting. If using a clot-activator tube, invert carefully 5–6 times to mix clot activator and blood before incubation.
9. Centrifuge for 15 min at 400 × $g$ at 4 °C. Do not use brake to stop centrifuge.
10. Carefully aspirate the supernatant (serum) at room temperature and pool into a centrifuge tube, taking care not to disturb the cell layer or transfer any cells. Use a clean pipette for each tube.
11. Inspect serum for turbidity. Turbid samples should be centrifuged and aspirated again to remove the remaining insoluble matter.
12. Aliquot into cryo-vials and store at −80 °C for the later analysis.

## 4 Notes

1. The entire process including isolation, purification, and transfer of the cells requires approx. 3–4 h. Typically, manifestation of inflammation will develop within 5–10 weeks following the cell transfer.
2. Analysis of the inflammation will be judged by MEICS score (murine endoscopic index of colitis severity). This will recognize five parameters (translucency, granularity, fibrin, vascularity, and stool) and will give a good survey [8, 9].
3. For the evaluation of the colon histopathology a blind-folded analysis gives the optimal results. This should be scored with respect of the following parameters (mucosal erosion and ulceration process, loss of crypt architecture, submucosal spread and transmural involvement, loss of goblet cells, and infiltration of neutrophils) [10]. In brief, the lowest grade should be given when there were no changes observed. Changes typically associated with other grades are as follows: grade 1 is associated with minimal scattered mucosal inflammatory cell infiltrates, with or without minimal epithelial hyperplasia. Grade 2 is given when a mild scattered to diffuse inflammatory cell infiltrates, sometimes extending into the submucosa and associated with erosions, with minimal to mild epithelial hyperplasia and minimal to mild mucin depletion from goblet cells are observed. A grade 3 is a mild-to-moderate inflammatory cell infiltrates, sometimes transmural and often associated with ulceration, with moderate epithelial hyperplasia and mucin depletion. Grade 4 is linked with a marked inflammatory cell infiltrates that were often transmural and associated with ulceration, with a marked epithelial hyperplasia and mucin depletion. Finally, grade 5 is given when a marked transmural inflammation with severe ulceration, loss of intestinal glands, and massive infiltration of neutrophils can be stated.

## 5 Troubleshooting

1. The injection of T-cells with lower cell viability causes in most cases a non-reconstitution of the immunodeficient recipient mice and no inflammation will be seen. Viability of the cells can be tested by counting the cells with Trypan blue staining and alternatively by fluorescent nucleic dye in FACS, like propidium iodide (PI) or 7-amino-actinomycin D (7-AAD). These dyes will be taken up by dead cells and consequently cells can be easily discriminated from living cells.

2. The injection of T-cells with a lower purity causes lower reconstitution of the immunodeficient recipient mice. It may be that mice get signs of inflammation later than normally or no inflammation will be obtained. To avoid this, do not inject cells with a purity of <98 %.
3. Sometimes, no inflammation will be seen when the technique of the i.p. injection is not done correctly. Then the cell suspension will be injected subcutaneously instead of intraperitoneally. In this case the cells are lost and no inflammation can be seen. To check this, isolate cells from spleen and analyze $CD4^+$ T-cells in FACS for reconstitution effort. If no or less T-cells can be found then mice are not to be reconstituted and no inflammation is visible.
4. The intestinal gut flora of the recipient mice is also important. The development of inflammation is additionally dependent on an intact bacterial flora. No antibiotics or acid-enriched drinking water should be administered to the mice. For best results a non-autoclaved food and a normal housing environment are advisable.
5. The choice of the recipient mice is dependent on the genetic background of the donor mice. If donor mice are on MHCII H-$2^b$ background then you can use (recombinase-activating gene) RAG-1- or RAG-2-deficient recipient mice. If donor mice are on MHCII H-$2^d$ background, then you should use (severe combined immunodeficiency) SCID or (non-obese diabetic/severe combined immunodeficiency) NOD-SCID or even NOD-SCID-IL-2Rγ KO mice for the transfer model. The advantage of using NOD-SCID or NOD-SCID-IL-2Rγ KO mice is that these mice have even a lower NK-cell activity and additionally impaired T-cell development functions, which may induce inflammation signs earlier.

## Acknowledgements

This work was supported by DFG grants WE46561/1, WE4656/2-1, and ELAN M1-09.06.23.1.

### References

1. Podolsky DK (2002) Inflammatory bowel disease. N Engl J Med 347(6):417–429
2. Elson CO, Cong Y, McCracken VJ, Dimmitt RA, Lorenz RG, Weaver CT (2005) Experimental models of inflammatory bowel disease reveal innate, adaptive, and regulatory mechanisms of host dialogue with the microbiota. Immunol Rev 206:260–276
3. Peluso I, Pallone F, Monteleone G (2006) Interleukin-12 and Th1 immune response in Crohn's disease: pathogenetic relevance and therapeutic implication. World J Gastroenterol 12(35):5606–5610
4. Monteleone G, Trapasso F, Parrello T, Biancone L, Stella A, Iuliano R, Luzza F, Fusco A, Pallone F (1999) Bioactive IL-18 expression is

up-regulated in Crohn's disease. J Immunol 163(1):143–147

5. Wirtz S, Neurath MF (2000) Animal models of intestinal inflammation: new insights into the molecular pathogenesis and immunotherapy of inflammatory bowel disease. Int J Colorectal Dis 15(3):144–160
6. Powrie F, Coffman RL, Correa-Oliveira R (1994) Transfer of CD4⁺ T cells to C.B-17 SCID mice: a model to study Th1 and Th2 cell differentiation and regulation in vivo. Res Immunol 145(5):347–353
7. Powrie F, Leach MW, Mauze S, Menon S, Caddle LB, Coffman RL (1994) Inhibition of Th1 responses prevents inflammatory bowel disease in scid mice reconstituted with $CD45RB^{hi}$ $CD4^{+}$ T cells. Immunity 1(7):553–556
8. Becker C, Fantini MC, Wirtz S, Nikolaev A, Kiesslich R, Lehr HA, Galle PR, Neurath MF (2005) In vivo imaging of colitis and colon cancer development in mice using high resolution chromoendoscopy. Gut 54(7): 950–954
9. Wirtz S, Becker C, Blumberg R, Galle PR, Neurath MF (2002) Treatment of T cell-dependent experimental colitis in SCID mice by local administration of an adenovirus expressing IL-18 antisense mRNA. J Immunol 168(1):411–420
10. Asseman C, Mauze S, Leach MW, Coffman RL, Powrie F (1999) An essential role for interleukin 10 in the function of regulatory T cells that inhibit intestinal inflammation. J Exp Med 190(7):995–1004

# Chapter 15

# Manipulation of T Cell Function and Conditional Gene Targeting in T Cells

Anna Śledzińska, Lynsey Fairbairn, and Thorsten Buch

## Abstract

Cre-Lox recombination is known as a site-specific recombinase technology, and is widely used to carry out modification at specific sites in the DNA of cells. The system consists of an enzyme, Cre recombinase, that recombines a pair of short target sequences, the *lox* sites. The Cre-Lox system can be used to activate or repress a gene depending on the placement of the *lox* sites. Placing the Cre recombinase under the control of a cell-specific promoter allows expression only in specific cells or cellular subsets, thus providing a powerful tool for analysis of gene function at specific developmental or physiological niches. Nowadays almost every aspect of T cell biology can be approached by a specific Cre model. This powerful tool allows scientists to overcome the limitations of gene-deficient animals and target a gene of interest specifically in T cell or T cell subsets by appropriate placement of the *lox* sites. Here we describe the main Cre lines that enable gene targeting in T helper cells or CD4 T cell subsets, and the most common methods of assessing the recombination efficiency.

**Key words** Cre-mediated recombination, Cre recombinase, Tamoxifen-inducible CreER$^{t2}$ system, Tamoxifen, Tamoxifen citrate chow

## 1 Introduction

### 1.1 Conditional Mutagenesis

Studies of gene function in the context of the whole organism have been radically advanced by generation of genetically mutant mice. Homologous integration of a targeting vector into the genome of murine embryonic stem cells (ES) allows sequence-specific alterations. Such novel mouse lines carry predesigned mutations, for instance gene deletions, insertions, or point mutations. Although this method has proven to be tremendously successful, it also suffers from some restrictions. For example some gene deficiencies are lethal during embryonic development and thus preclude the study of gene function in the mature organism. In other instances it is of particular interest to study the role of a gene in a defined developmental stage, or the function of a particular cell type, an analysis that is generally not possible in a traditional gene-deficient animal.

Ari Waisman and Burkhard Becher (eds.), *T-Helper Cells: Methods and Protocols*, Methods in Molecular Biology, vol. 1193, DOI 10.1007/978-1-4939-1212-4_15, © Springer Science+Business Media New York 2014

Traditional transgenesis allows only the study of inherited genetic disorders and not conditions which have an environmental component like cancer. These shortcomings have been overcome by the development of conditional mutagenic models in which sequences of interest, flanked by target sites of a recombinase, are removed by a separately expressed recombinase. The most commonly used recombinase for such purposes is the Cre recombinase from the bacteriophage P1. It recognizes the 34 bp long *loxP* site consisting of two 13 bp long palindromic sequences separated by an 8 bp long nonpalindromic spacer that gives orientation to the site. The *loxP* site is small enough to be considered as a neutral sequence when inserted in the genome, but is also long enough to be specific within the mouse genome. *LoxP* sites of similar direction that flank a sequence, called a "floxed" sequence, will lead to the removal of the intervening sequence segment; *loxP* sites of opposite direction will lead to its inversion. By appropriate positioning of the two *loxP* sites this system of mutagenesis can produce deletions, insertions, and point mutations. The combination of transgenically expressed Cre recombinase and a *loxP*-flanked gene (or a segment thereof) has become a powerful tool that enables researchers to overcome the described limitations of gene-deficient animals. One mouse line carries the Cre recombinase under the control of a specific promoter, so that the Cre activity is restricted to a defined tissue or cell line. Another line carries the floxed gene. When the two strains are bred together, the floxed gene is modified in the offspring only in cells which express Cre. With this approach, the function of different genes can be studied in a cell line or a tissue of interest. Further improvement of the system has been achieved by fusing Cre to a mutant of the ligand-binding domain of the estrogen receptor (ER), which allows the recombinase to be inducible by administration of tamoxifen. This chimeric protein, usually an ER mutant with higher affinity for tamoxifen and lower affinity for β-estradiol (CreER$^{t2}$), remains located in the cytoplasm unless its activator tamoxifen is present. Only when tamoxifen binds to the ER portion of the fusion protein is the heat-shock protein HSP90 released and the Cre fusion molecule enters the nucleus, where it catalyzes the recombination of the floxed DNA sequence. Thus, CreER$^{t2}$ allows the researcher to control Cre activity in a temporal manner and induce gene modifications at a defined time point.

### 1.2 T Cell-Specific Conditional Mutagenesis

Conditional mutagenesis within the T cell lineage has been of great success and yielded a large number of new insights into the biology of this cell type. By now almost every aspect of T cell development and differentiation as well as function can be approached by a specific Cre model. Thymic development is frequently analyzed through combination of Vav-Cre, Lck-Cre (lymphocyte protein tyrosine kinase), and CD4-Cre. The Vav-Cre-mediated recombination is not specific for T cell progenitors and occurs in many hematopoietic cells. To target the gene of interest in the early thymic developmental stage ($CD4^-CD8^-$), the transgenic line expressing Cre under the proximal Lck promoter can be used. CD4-Cre, known as one of the most efficient Cre lines, enables recombination in the double-positive ($CD4^+CD8^+$) stage of thymocyte development. To summarize Cre-dependent recombination occurs before positive selection in the thymus in all of these lines, and this is also true for *hCD2-icre* mice. Combining the data generated from experiments using these Cre strains on the same loxP-flanked target allele allows the determination of the role of the gene during the specific phases of development. This will also allow circumvention of possible blocks as a result of the absence of the gene in an earlier stage, which would otherwise have precluded the analysis of the cell population of interest.

The Cre-mediated recombination through the Vav, Lck, and CD4-Cre lines will subsequently result in recombination in $CD4^+$ and $CD8^+$ postthymic T cells. Consequently it is difficult to distinguish if the phenotype observed after deletion/induction of the gene of interest is the result of perturbed thymic development or if the gene is also crucial for mature T cell homeostasis and function. To avoid affecting thymic development and focus on which role the gene of interest may play in mature T cells, Cre lines that recombine in mature T cells can be used. The dLck-Cre (distal-Lck) strain allows gene modification in positively selected thymocytes and T cells, excluding regulatory T cells. The exact timing of this Cre-mediated recombination is, however, unclear. On the basis of the expression of reporter protein (*see* Table 1) the efficiency of dLck-Cre-mediated recombination was high reaching 75 % in $CD4^+$ T cells and >90 % in $CD8^+$ T cells. OX40-Cre can be used to assess the role of a gene of interest for activated ($CD44^{hi}$) T cells. In contrast to dLck-Cre, OX40-Cre is also active in regulatory ($Foxp3^+$) $CD4^+$ T cells but allows only minor recombination in activated $CD8^+$ T cells. Moreover defined T cell subsets, such as Th17 cells and regulatory T cells, can be targeted using specific Cre recombinases, IL-17-Cre and Foxp3-Cre, respectively. Two separate Cre lines have been generated to modify the target gene expression in Th17 cells: IL-17A-Cre and IL-17F-Cre (Table 1). Both Cre lines were crossed to ROSA-EYFP reporter strains for initial analysis and expression of fluorescent protein was shown to correlate with the expression of the IL-17 cytokine. In addition IL-17-Cre strains crossed to reporter strains can be used to map the fate of IL-17-expressing T cells. Foxp3-Cre strain is a convenient tool for gene manipulation in regulatory T cells (Table 1). Additionally the Cre in this strain was fused to YFP reporter protein and its expression was confirmed to correlate with Foxp3 expression. Furthermore, new mouse models allow induced recombination in the T cell subsets through application of tamoxifen. These include $CD4\text{-}CreER^{t2}$ generated in our laboratory and

**Table 1**
**Cre strains that can mediate gene modifications in T cells**

| Short name | ILAR-assigned registration code | Recombine cell type | Cre fused with fluorescent protein | References |
|---|---|---|---|---|
| Lck-Cre | B6. Cg-TgN(LckCre)548Jxm | DN thymocytes<br>DP thymocytes<br>CD4 SP thymocytes<br>CD8 SP thymocytes<br>CD4$^+$ T cells<br>CD8$^+$ T cells | No | Hennet T et al. (1995) PNAS<br>Orban PC et al. (1992) PNAS<br>Lee PP et al. (2001) Immunity |
| *CD2Cre* (*hCD2-iCre*) | B6.Cg-Tg (CD2-cre)4Kio/J | T and B cell precursors<br>T cells and B cells | No | Zhumabekov T et al. (1995) J Imm Methods<br>Shimshek DR et al. (2002) Genesis<br>De Boer J et al. (2003) Eur J Immunol |
| RORc-Cre | B6. FVB-Tg(Rorc-cre)1Litt/J<br>C57BL/6-Tg(rorc-cre)Lit | DP thymocytes<br>CD4 SP thymocytes<br>CD8 SP thymocytes<br>CD4$^+$ T cells<br>CD8$^+$ T cells<br>Subset of ILCs | No<br>Crossed to GFP reporter | Eberl G and Littman D (2004) Science |
| Vav-Cre | B6.Cg-Tg(Vav1-cre) A2Kio/J | Majority of hematopoietic and endothelial cells | No | Pantelis G et al. (2002) Genesis |
| CD4-Cre | B6.Cg-Tg(Cd4-cre)1Cwi/ BfluJ<br>B6.Cg-Tg(CD4-cre)1Cwi | DP thymocytes<br>CD4 SP thymocytes<br>CD8 SP thymocytes<br>CD4$^+$ T cells<br>CD8$^+$ T cells | No | Lee PP et al. (2001) Immunity<br>Wolfer A et al. (2001) Nat Imm |
| dLck-Cre | B6. Cg-Tg(Lck-cre)3779Nik/J | Postthymic CD4$^+$ T and CD8$^+$ T cells | No | Wang Q et al. (2001) J Exp Med<br>Zhang DJ et al. (2005) J Immunol |

(continued)

**Table 1 (continued)**

| Short name | ILAR-assigned registration code | Recombine cell type | Cre fused with fluorescent protein | References |
|---|---|---|---|---|
| OX40-Cre | B6.129X1(Cg)-Tnfrsf4$^{tm2(cre)Nik}$/J *B6.Cg-Tnfrsf4$^{tm2(cre)Nik}$/J* | Regulatory T cells Activated CD4$^{+}$ T cells (memory/memory-like phenotype) Low expression in activated CD8$^{+}$ T cells | No Bred to ROSA-YFP reporter strains | Klinger M et al. (2009) J Immunol |
| Foxp3-Cre | B6.129(Cg)-Foxp3$^{tm4(YFP/cre)Ayr}$/J | Foxp3-expressing regulatory T cells | Yes, YFP | Rubstov YP et al. (2008) Immunity |
| IL-17F-Cre | B6-Tg(Il17f-cre)1Awai | Th17 cells IL-17-producing CD8$^{+}$ T cells | No, crossed with ROSA-eYFP reporter | Croxford A et al. (2009) J Immunol |
| IL-17A-Cre | Il17a$^{tm1.1(icre)Stck}$/J (129×1/SvJ x 129S1/Sv) F1-Kitl<+> | Th17 cells IL-17-producing CD8$^{+}$ T cells IL-17-producing ILCs | No, crossed with ROSA-eYFP reporter | Hirota K et al. (2011) Nat Imm |
| CD4-CreER$^{t2}$ | B6-CD4<tm1(CreER$^{t2}$) ThBu | Depends on tamoxifen treatment regime and the target gene Postthymic CD4$^{+}$ T cells DP thymocytes—low recombination SP CD4 thymocytes—low recombination SP CD8 thymocytes—low recombination | No | Sledzinska A et al. (2013) PLOS Biology |
| Foxp3-Cre-ERt2 | Foxp3$^{tm9(EGFP/cre/ERT2)Ayr}$/J | After tamoxifen treatment Foxp3-expressing regulatory T cells | Yes, EGFP | Rubstov YP et al. (2010) Science |

Foxp3-CreER$^{t2}$ strains. The CD4CreER$^{t2}$ mouse allows efficient recombination in postthymic CD4$^{+}$, but not in CD8$^{+}$ T cells. In contrast to conventional CD4-Cre, the tamoxifen-inducible model allows only low-level recombination in the DP stage of thymic development. The Foxp3-CreER$^{t2}$ mouse can be used to target genes of interest in regulatory T cells after tamoxifen treatment. This construct, similar to Foxp3-Cre, contains fluorescent reporter protein (EGFP) fused to a CreER$^{t2}$. These mice may then be useful for studying lineage stability and genetic mapping of regulatory T cells.

### 1.3 Analysis of Recombination Efficiency

Information about the extent of the Cre-mediated recombination is a crucial and often somewhat neglected aspect of studies involving conditional mutagenesis. It should be stressed that if recombination for one floxed target allele has been reported to be specific and efficient, an identical outcome cannot be readily assumed when using a different target allele. Recombination of a new allele may take place in a broader number of cell types or the frequency may be drastically lower while the specificity is retained. Every study should therefore start with a thorough analysis of the recombination frequency. It may nevertheless help to first establish a novel Cre system by indirect assays, such as provided by reporter lines. Thus, many Cre lines (e.g., IL-17F-Cre, CD4-CreER$^{t2}$, or OX40-Cre) (Table 1) were crossed to reporter strains for initial characterization. Some Cre mice have also been engineered to co-express a reporter protein with the recombinase (Table 1). While this setup allows the easy identification of recombinase-positive cells, it will not yield any information about recombination per se. In many cases the expression of a reporter protein, e.g., GFP or YFP, can be measured by flow cytometry. As already mentioned recombination depends highly on the organization and chromosomal structure of the target allele. Thus, the extent of recombination estimated by the expression of reporter protein may not necessarily apply to the research target. It is therefore recommended to assess deletion or induction of respective proteins for each target allele separately. As an example the CD4Cre-ER$^{t2}$ mouse was crossed to TGF-βRII$^{fl/fl}$ strain and ROSA/EYFP reporter strain. Upon tamoxifen application around 90 % of CD4$^{+}$ T cells had TGF-βRII deleted; however only 21 % of CD4$^{+}$ T cells were positive for EYFP and negative for TGF-βRII (Fig. 1).

The deletion or the overexpression of the protein by CD4$^{+}$ T cells can be determined directly by FACS analysis if the specific antibody is available. It is recommended to include additional antibodies to distinguish between different CD4$^{+}$ T cell subsets like naïve, effector/effector memory, or regulatory cells in the staining panels. These will allow confirmation of equal deletion in all subsets as expected for, e.g., CD4-Cre or CD4Cre-ER$^{t2}$ strains.

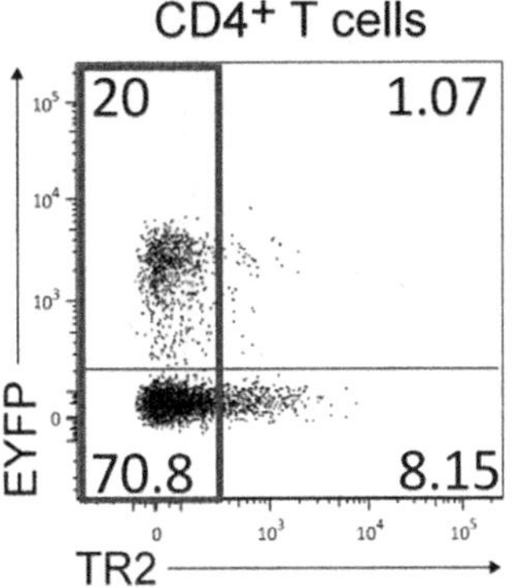


**Fig. 1** Flow cytometric analysis of TGF-βRII (TR2) and EYFP expression by CD4$^+$ T cells isolated from CD4CreER$^{t2}$ x TGF-βRII$^{fl/fl}$ x ROSA/EYFP mouse strain 2 weeks post-tamoxifen application

It is also necessary to perform additional intracellular staining for Cre strains that are designed to recombine only in certain subsets like IL-17-Cre of Foxp3-Cre. Western blot analysis can be used as an alternative to flow cytometry. One primary advantage of using Western blotting in preference to flow cytometric analysis is the far greater number of antibodies available. Western blotting can be performed on protein lysate isolated from purified CD4$^+$ T cells or CD4$^+$ T cell subsets, but requires time-consuming cell sorting and does not provide single-cell information. If the antibody is not available or the expression of the gene of interest at the protein level is too low to perform quantitative analysis, real-time quantitative PCR (RT qPCR) is another possibility. To assess gene expression at the mRNA instead of protein level, a pair of primers can be designed such that at least one primer is located in the sequence removed by the recombination event. Similarly, RT qPCR can be used for detection of induced gene expression subsequent to a recombination event. Theoretically quantitative genomic PCR can also be used to assess recombination, but care has to be taken regarding normalization. Moreover due to the usually higher ratio of mRNA to the encoding gene, any effect is easier to detect by RT qPCR. While Southern blot analysis is still the gold standard for identification of homologous recombination events, its daily use for quantification of Cre-mediated recombination has waned in the recent years. Finally a point of caution must be made when using any of the methods which do not involve single-cell analysis (such as Western blot, qRT-PCR, Southern blot). In case of a certain detected recombination frequency, for example 50 %, it is not clear whether all cells have recombined only one allele, or half the cells have recombined both alleles (or some variable in between). In such cases it may be useful to assess the outcome of recombination at the functional level. To investigate if the ablation of the cytokine receptor expressed by $CD4^+$ T cells was efficient stimulation was subsequently used as readout. As an example $CD4^+$ T cells isolated from either CD4-Cre or $CD4Cre^{Er,t2}$ TGF-$\beta RII^{fl/fl,\ fl/Fl}$ mice can be stimulated with TGF-β and phosphorylation of Smad2 or -3 investigated by Western blot. Likewise impaired phosphorylation of STAT transcription factors will indicate efficient deletion of cytokine receptor deletion and can be assessed by flow cytometry or Western blot analysis. The ablation of the transcription factor involved in certain cytokine production in T helper cells, e.g., RORγt, can be determined by skewing $CD4^+$ T cells into Th17 cells and measuring the production of IL-17 either by Intracellular Staining Cytokines and Transcription Factors (*see* chap. 5) or by ELISA.

In the end, the assay chosen depends on the floxed target gene and is thus specific to the scientific project.

## 2 Materials

### 2.1 Induction of CreER$^{t2}$ System In Vivo

1. Tamoxifen.
2. Corn oil (or olive oil, peanut oil).
3. Ethanol (96 %).
4. Vortex.
5. Sonicator or ultrasonic bath.
6. Balance.
7. Heating block (or water bath).
8. Syringes/needles:
   (a) For i.p. 25G5/8 needles.
   (b) 1 ml syringe with luer-lock (dependent on the gavage needle).
   (c) Gavage needle (feeding needles bent or straight, gauge 18).
9. Tamoxifen citrate food and respective control food.

### 2.2 Induction of CreER$^{t2}$ System In Vitro

1. 4-Hydroxytamoxifen.
2. Ethanol (99 %).
3. PBS (pH 7.4).
4. RPMI 1640 medium complete (RPMI medium supplemented with 10 % FCS, 1 % penicillin-streptomycin, 0.5 % 2-mercaptoethanol).
5. Optional depending on the assay: Anti-CD3 antibody, anti-CD28 antibody.
6. Standard laboratory equipment including cell culture dishes, 70 μm nylon cell strainers, 50 ml sterile tubes, pipettes.
7. Laminar flow, incubators.

#### 2.3 Analysis of Deletion Efficiency

##### 2.3.1 Southern Blot

1. Agarose gel 0.7 % with Et-Br, DNA ladder.
2. Gel chamber, combs, gel tray.
3. Digested DNA (samples).
4. Buffers:
   (a) TAE buffer (tris-acetate-EDTA buffer): Composition of 50× TAE buffer: 2.0 M Tris–HCl acetate, 0.05 M EDTA, pH 8.2–8.4.
   (b) 0.25 M HCl, 0.4 M NaOH.
   (c) Transfer solutions: 0.4 M NaOH, 0.6 M NaCl (should be freshly prepared).
   (d) Neutralization buffers: 0.5 M Tris–HCl (pH 7), 0.6 M NaCl.
   (e) Hybridization solution:

| | |
|---|---|
| 1 M NaCl | 59 g NaCl |
| 50 mM Tris–HCl pH 7.5 | 50 ml 1 M Tris–HCl |
| 10 % Dextran sulfate | 100 g |
| 1 % SDS | 100 ml 10 % SDS solution |
| Salmon sperm DNA (sonicated): | 25 ml 10 mg/ml solution |
| Fill up to 800 ml, dissolve at 65 °C | |
| Fill to 1,000 ml, and freeze 30 ml aliquots | |

| |
|---|
| 20× SSC (saline-sodium citrate buffer): For 1 L pH: 7 (add five drops of 37 % HCl to adjust pH) |
| NaCl 175.3 g end cc.: 3 M |
| Na citrate (trisodium citrate) 88.2 g end cc.: 0.3 M |

5. Probes, random primers, water, Bca buffer, dNTPs, Bca polymerase for PCR reaction.
6. Paper towels, Whatman paper, nylon membrane.
7. Column, safe-lock tube.
8. Hybridization oven, heating block, vortex.

##### 2.3.2 PCR and Real-Time qPCR (RT qPCR)

PCR

1. Primer mix (10 μM each, concentration to be determined by the user).
2. Template DNA.
3. DNA polymerase (e.g., Taq polymerase).
4. PCR buffer (with or without Mg).
5. $MgCl_2$ or $Mg_2SO_4$ (depends on the buffer)
6. RNase-free, DNase-free water.
7. PCR thermal cycler.

8. Agarose gel, DNA ladder.
9. Gel chamber, combs.

Real-Time qPCR

1. mRNA isolated from sorted $CD4^+$ T cells or $CD4^+$ T cell subset.
2. Polymerase reverse transcriptase (e.g., Moloney murine leukemia virus (M-MLV) transcriptase).
3. Oligo (dT) or random primers.
4. dNTPs.
5. Buffer—specific to the polymerase.
6. cDNA (template DNA).
7. Primers designed for the transcript of interest and housekeeping gene (ideal amplicon size should be between 80 and 200 b.p.).
8. DNA polymerase.
9. Molecular biology-grade water, RNase free (commercially available or DEPC treated).
10. Reference dye.
11. Pipettes, PCR, tubes, 96- or 384-well plate (depends on cycler).
12. Heating block or thermal cycler, real-time PCR cycler.

## 3 Methods

### 3.1 Induction of CreER$^{t2}$ In Vivo

#### 3.1.1 Preparation of Tamoxifen/Oil Emulsion for Gavage and i.p. Treatment

Tamoxifen is light sensitive. Therefore overexposure to strong light should be avoided.

If not stated otherwise, the whole procedure is conducted at room temperature.

Solubility: Tamoxifen in ethanol approximately 20 mg/ml.

(*A*) *Preparation of oil/tamoxifen emulsion*:

1. Weigh 100 mg of tamoxifen powder and add 100 µl of 96 % ethanol to reach a final concentration of 1 g/ml.
2. Vortex the suspension for 10–15 min. (Note: In this concentration it is not possible to dissolve all of the tamoxifen in ethanol.)
3. Add 900 µl of corn oil (or other kinds of oil) to obtain a final concentration of 100 mg/ml to the tamoxifen/ethanol suspension. Vortex thoroughly and incubate for 15 min at 56 °C in heat block shaking or water bath, preferably with shaking.
4. After this procedure some crystals might still be visible. To obtain a homogenous suspension sonicate briefly in a sonic bath (such as used to clean tools). Repeat until no crystals remain visible. Aliquots can be stored at −20 °C. Avoid multiple freeze-thaw cycles.

(*B*) *Oral treatment with tamoxifen/oil by gavage*:

The exact dose of tamoxifen as well as the treatment regime should be determined empirically depending on the purpose of the experiment, the target gene, and the age of the animal. To achieve maximal recombination in CD4$^+$ T cells, apply tamoxifen through gavage for 5–8 consecutive days or every second day when longer treatment is required (*see* **Note 1**). For induction of genes (or targets that recombine easily) a single gavage can be sufficient. Both methods, application once and for 5 days, have allowed our laboratory to perform pulse-chase experiments.

1. Thaw aliquots of tamoxifen/oil and place at 37 °C. No crystals should be visible and the solution should be homogenous.
2. Use 1 ml luer-lock syringe and gavage needle. Perform the oral treatment of the mice according to standard procedures.
3. Feed mouse with 5 mg tamoxifen (50 μl; around 200 mg tamoxifen per 1 kg body weight) for 5 consecutive days.
4. Observe mice every day for behavior/health indicative of stress, discomfort, or disease. If any pathological changes are observed titrate further the amount of tamoxifen used.

(*C*) *Intraperitoneal injection of tamoxifen*:

The amount of tamoxifen required for efficient Cre-mediated recombination but which is still safe for the animals should be determined empirically. Start with approximately 75 mg tamoxifen/kg body weight applied in 100 μl [1].

1. Thaw aliquots of tamoxifen solution in oil and pre-warm at 37 °C. No crystals should be visible and the solution should be homogenous.
2. Perform the i.p. injection according to standard procedure.
3. Repeat up to five times on consecutive days.
4. Observe mice daily for behavior/health indicative of stress, discomfort, or disease. Titrate down the amount of tamoxifen if any pathological changes are observed.

#### 3.1.2 Tamoxifen Citrate Chow

Feeding of the experimental animals with chow containing tamoxifen citrate is the method of choice when long-term deletion is required. The frequency of Cre-mediated recombination should be tested at several time points during the long-term tamoxifen treatment. We observed that the time to achieve efficient recombination with tamoxifen citrate chow appears longer than with i.p. injection or gavage, possibly because daily doses of uptake are lower.

Use the mouse food pellets with 400 mg/kg tamoxifen. Feed the animals for 1–5 weeks with tamoxifen pellets or control food. Do not forget to order the control food with the tamoxifen food. In most animal facilities it will differ from the regular chow. Observe animals for behavior/health changes indicative of stress, discomfort, or disease throughout the experiment. The mice may lose weight temporarily after switching to the tamoxifen citrate diet. Depending on the ingredients of the tamoxifen food pellets the mice may not gain as much weight as with standard food [2]. This should be taken into consideration when changes in body weight are the readout of the experiment.

### 3.2 Induction of the CreER$^{t2}$ System In Vitro

While the main purpose of inducible Cre systems is the in vivo analysis of gene function, it is nevertheless sometimes useful to induce the recombination in vitro. This can allow, for example, the recombination to take place during in vitro T cell differentiation assays. To achieve Cre-mediated recombination in vitro it is recommended to use 4-hydroxytamoxifen, a water-soluble, active metabolite of tamoxifen.

1. Prepare 4-hydroxytamoxifen aliquots: Dissolve 4-hydroxytamoxifen in ethanol to obtain 5 mM (1.94 mg/ml). Store aliquots at −20 °C and protect from the light.
2. Prepare RPMI 1640 complete medium. Isolate lymphocytes from spleen or lymph nodes of CreER$^{t2}$-positive and control mice according to standard procedure. Place the cells in culture with RPMI 1640 complete medium at a concentration of $4 \times 10^6$ cells/ml medium. Different concentrations of the ligand should be tested in the range of 0.1–5 μM (end concentration). Dependent on the experimental design, recombination in combination with activation of the T cells may also be tested. So the following conditions can be tested:
   (a) No activation.
   (b) Stimulation with anti-CD3 (5 μg/ml) and anti-CD28 (2 μg/ml) antibody (please *see* **Note 2**).
   (c) Stimulation with PMA and ionomycin.
   (d) Polarizing condition (i.e., anti-CD3 and anti-CD28 stimulation with addition of cytokines).
3. Maintain the cells in the 4-hydroxytamoxifen for 3–5 days depending on the experiment. If it is necessary to keep cells in culture longer, wash the cells after 5 days and add fresh medium with 4-hydroxytamoxifen; 4-hydroxytamoxifen can undergo cis-trans interconversion in culture media.

### 3.3 Assessing Deletion Efficiency

#### 3.3.1 Southern Blot Analysis

1. Pour 0.7 % agarose gel with ethidium bromide. Add loading buffer to the digested DNA samples. Load DNA and the size marker into the pockets.
2. Start the run of the gel at 80 V for 2 min. Run overnight at 40–50 V.

3. Take the picture of the gel, and mark the size ladder by punching little holes into the gel (e.g., with a 20–200 μl tip).
4. Shake gel carefully in 0.25 M HCl no longer than 15 min.
5. Shake gel in 0.4 M NaOH for 15 min.

   Transfer:

6. Place two 5 cm stacks of paper towels next to each other and on top of the paper place two wet Whatman papers, slightly larger than the gel, wet with transfer buffer.
7. Wet the membrane with transfer buffer and place it on the Whatman paper; avoid bubbles by rolling a 10 ml pipette over the stack.
8. Place two wet Whatman papers on the gel.
9. Build a bridge of Whatman paper (two layers) to a reservoir with transfer buffer. Transfer for at least 4 h or overnight.
10. When disassembling the blot do not forget to mark the ladder on the membrane with a pencil.
11. Neutralize membrane in neutralization buffer for 10 min—0.5 M Tris–HCl (pH 7) and 0.6 M NaCl.
12. Bake membrane between Whatman paper at 65–70 °C in a hybridization oven for 1 h.
13. Blot can be stored dry at RT.
14. Pre-wet membrane with 2× SSC and then incubate in 15–20 ml of prehyb/hyb solution overnight (or for at least 2 h) at 65 °C in rotator.

    Labelling of the probe:

15. Label probe, add it to hybridization solution, and rotate overnight at 65 °C. For probe purification use low-melting agarose from PCR reactions.
16. Prepare the reaction mixture in safe-lock tubes. Add 2 μl of the random primers and 50–1,000 ng of probe. The total volume should be 16.5 μl, and adjust with water.
17. Place the reaction mixture in boiling water for 3 min and then place the tube on ice for 5 min.
18. Add 2.5 μl Bca buffer and 2.5 μl random primers and 1 μl Bca polymerase to the reaction mix. From now on the procedure must be conducted in a laboratory certified for use of radioisotopes according to the safety instruction.
19. Add 2.5 μl $P^{32}$-CTP to the reaction mixture, to obtain end volume of 25 μl.
20. Incubate the reaction mix in 50 °C for 30 min to 1 h. Add 100 μl of $H_2O$ to the reaction mix.

21. Prepare the column by vortexing and centrifuging according to the manufacturer's protocol.
22. Place column into a tube, add reaction mix, centrifuge, and compare counts in column to counts in probe (should be 50 % in each).
23. Place in boiling water for 3 min, use *safe-lock tube,* and then on ice for 5 min.
24. Add to the pre-hybridization solution but never directly to the membrane.
25. Rotate overnight at 65 °C.
26. Wash membrane twice with 2× SSC buffer at 65 °C; counts should be around 200–500 cpm. Stringency of washing can be increased by using 1× and 0.5× SSC and addition of 1 % final concentration of SDS. The washing conditions have to be determined empirically.
27. Place the membrane in plastic bag, seal, and read the radiation with a phosphor screen.

### 3.3.2 PCR and Real-Time qPCR (RT qPCR) Analysis

*Primer design—a general note*:
In general, probe sequence should be free of secondary structure and should not hybridize to themselves or to primer 3′ ends. The optimal concentration of probe may vary between 50 and 800 nM, with a recommended starting concentration of 100 nM. PCR primers used with probes should be designed according to standard PCR guidelines. They should be specific for the target sequence and free of internal secondary structure, and should avoid complementation at 3′ ends within each primer, with each other, or with the dual-labeled probe. Optimal results may require a titration of primer concentrations between 100 and 500 nM. A final concentration of 200 nM per primer is effective for most reactions. The primers for assessing the efficiency recombination efficiency should be designed in the way that at least one of them binds to the floxed exon.

#### PCR

Different DNA polymerases can be used depending on the specific experimental conditions and protocol. Taq polymerase is one of the most commonly used but the manufacturer's instructions specific to the polymerase used should always be consulted. The following basic protocol serves as a general guideline and a starting point for any PCR amplification. Optimal reaction conditions (incubation times and temperatures, concentration of *Taq* DNA polymerase, primers, $MgCl_2$, and template DNA) vary and need to be optimized.

1. PCR reactions should be assembled in a DNA-free environment. Use of "clean" dedicated automatic pipettes and

aerosol-resistant barrier tips is recommended. *Always* keep the control DNA and other templates to be amplified isolated from the other components.

2. Add the following components to a sterile 0.5 ml microcentrifuge tube sitting on ice:

| Components | Volume | Final concentration |
|---|---|---|
| 10× PCR buffer minus Mg | 10 μl | 1× |
| 10 mM dNTP mixture | 2 μl | 0.2 mM each |
| 50 mM $MgCl_2$ | 3 μl | 1.5 mM |
| Primer mix (10 μM each) | 5 μl | 0.5 μM each |
| Template DNA | 1–20 μl | n/a |
| *Taq* DNA polymerase (5 U/μl) | 0.5 μl | 2.5 units |
| RNase-free, DNase-free water | to 100 μl | n/a |

A master mix should be prepared for multiple reactions, to minimize reagent loss and enable accurate pipetting.

3. Optional: Mix contents of the tube and overlay with 50 μl of mineral or silicone oil.
4. Cap tubes and centrifuge briefly to collect the contents to the bottom.
5. Incubate tubes in a thermal cycler at 94 °C for 3 min to completely denature the template.
6. Perform 25–35 cycles of PCR amplification as follows:

| |
|---|
| Denature at 94 °C for 45 s |
| Anneal at X °C for 30 s |
| Extend at 72 °C for 1 min (estimate: 1 min per kb) |

7. Incubate for an additional 10 min at 72 °C and maintain the reaction at 10 °C. The samples can be stored at −20 °C until use.
8. Analyze the amplification products by agarose gel electrophoresis and visualize by ethidium bromide or alternative staining. Use appropriate molecular weight standards.

#### cDNA Synthesis (Reverse Transcription) and qPCR

Isolate mRNA from purified $CD4^+$ T cells or $CD4^+$ T cell subsets using standard molecular biology protocol or a commercially available kit. Measure concentration of RNA in the sample.

The protocol for synthesis of single-strand cDNA is as follows:

1. Take 1–5 μg total RNA in 10 μl RNase-free $H_2O$ per reaction.

2. Heat the sample to 65 °C for 5 min and then quench on ice.
3. Prepare the master mix for one reaction:

| |
|---|
| 1 μl random primers (100 ng/μl) |
| 1 μl dNTP (10 mM) |
| 4 μl PCR buffer (5×) |
| 2 μl DTT (0.1 M) |

4. Mix gently and incubate master mix for 2 min at 37 °C.
5. Add 1 μl M-MLV RT (200 U/μl) per reaction to the master mix, and mix gently by pipetting.
6. Give 10 μl of master mix to the RNA sample.
7. Incubate the reaction mix:

| |
|---|
| 10 min at room temperature |
| 50 min at 37 °C |
| 15 min at 70 °C |

The cDNA can now be used as a template for amplification in PCR. However, amplification of some PCR targets (>1 kb) may require the removal of RNA complementary to the cDNA.

*qPCR*:
There are two main detection methods for quantitating gene levels in "real time."

*Fluorescent DNA-binding dyes*:
Nonspecific fluorescent binding dyes, e.g., SYBR® Green, intercalate with double-stranded DNA and increases in fluorescence are monitored throughout the PCR cycle to provide quantification of relative amounts of double-stranded DNA.

*Fluorescently labeled probes*:
Primer sets that include one primer labeled with a single fluorophore and one corresponding unlabeled primer, e.g., LUX™, are also available for RT qPCR. Fluorescent dual-labeled probe technology such as TaqMan® probes is also commonly used. Dual-labeled probes use two PCR primers as well as a probe that hybridizes to the internal portion of the amplicon.

Individual manufacturer's protocols should be consulted for starting concentrations; in general all RT qPCR reactions will be 25 or 50 μl and should contain the following.

A master mix should be prepared for multiple reactions, to minimize reagent loss and enable accurate pipetting.

1. Mix contents of the tube and pipette appropriate volume into wells of a PCR plate.

2. Cap tubes and centrifuge briefly to collect the contents to the bottom.
3. Place tubes in thermal cycle and use appropriate program: *Example program*:

| 50 °C for 2 min |
|---|
| 95 °C for 10 min |
| Followed by 35–40 cycles |
| Denature at 94–95 °C for 5–15 s |
| Anneal at 55–60 °C for 30–60 s |
| Extend at 72 °C for 30–60 s |
| Melt curve analysis can be used to ensure that only a single product has been synthesized |
| Please consult your instrument software on how to generate a melt curve |

## 4 Notes

1. Check prior to the treatment the length of the gavage needle by measuring from the tip of the animal's head to the last rib (to avoid perforation of the stomach; important when smaller animals are fed).
2. If a pure population of $CD4^+$ T cells is taken into culture, it is necessary to coat the plate with anti-CD3 antibody prior to starting the culture. The co-stimulatory antibody (anti-CD28) can be either plate bound or soluble.

### References

1. Madisen L et al (2010) A robust and high-throughput Cre reporting and characterization system for the whole mouse brain. Nat Neurosci 13(1):133–40
2. Kiermayer C et al (2007) Optimization of spatio-temporal gene inactivation in mouse heart by oral application of tamoxifen citrate. Genesis 45(1): 11–6

# Chapter 16

# Aldara-Induced Psoriasis-Like Skin Inflammation: Isolation and Characterization of Cutaneous Dendritic Cells and Innate Lymphocytes

C.T. Wohn, S. Pantelyushin, J.L. Ober-Blöbaum, and B.E. Clausen

## Abstract

Psoriasis is a chronic auto-inflammatory skin disease of unknown etiology affecting millions of people worldwide. Dissecting the cellular networks and molecular signals promoting the development of psoriasis critically depends on appropriate animal models. Topical application of Aldara cream containing the Toll-like receptor (TLR)7-ligand Imiquimod induces skin inflammation and pathology in mice closely resembling plaque-type psoriasis in humans. The particular power of the Aldara model lies in examining the early events during psoriatic plaque formation, which is difficult to achieve in patients. Hence, recent reports using this model have challenged currently prevailing concepts concerning the pathophysiology of psoriasis. Here, we describe the induction and phenotype of Aldara-mediated dermatitis in mice and, in particular, analysis of the inflammatory cell infiltrate using flow cytometry.

**Key words** Aldara cream, Dendritic cells, γδ T cells, Imiquimod, Innate lymphocytes, Psoriasis, Psoriatic skin inflammation

## 1 Introduction

Plaque-type psoriasis is a common multifactorial inflammatory skin disease characterized by erythematous scaling skin lesions. Histologically psoriasis exhibits a thickened epidermis due to hyper-proliferation and disturbed differentiation of keratinocytes, together with leukocyte infiltrates mainly consisting of T cells, monocytes/macrophages, dendritic cells (DC), and neutrophils. Although the pathogenesis of psoriasis is not completely clear, it is probably provoked by environmental triggers in genetically predisposed individuals and involves both innate and adaptive components of the immune system. Currently, it is widely held that plasmacytoid DC (pDC), through secretion of type-I interferons (IFN-I), elicit an auto-inflammatory cascade leading to enhanced activation of T helper (Th) type 1 and Th17 cells. Th1-derived TNFα and IFNγ and production of IL-17 and IL-22 by Th17 cells

Ari Waisman and Burkhard Becher (eds.), *T-Helper Cells: Methods and Protocols*, Methods in Molecular Biology, vol. 1193, DOI 10.1007/978-1-4939-1212-4_16, © Springer Science+Business Media New York 2014

in turn drive keratinocyte proliferation, antimicrobial peptide production, and leukocyte recruitment, ultimately resulting in the formation of psoriatic plaques [1]. However, the type of immune cell(s) and cytokine(s) essential during, respectively, the initiation and progression of psoriasis remain elusive.

Understanding the complex cellular interactions and molecular pathways of chronic inflammatory diseases critically relies on relevant and easily accessible mouse models. In the absence of a naturally occurring disorder in laboratory animals mimicking the multi-faceted phenotype of psoriasis, numerous transgenic and xeno-transplantation models have shed light on specific aspects implicated in the pathophysiology and therapy of this skin disease [2]. Based on the clinical observation that treatment of patients for unrelated conditions with Aldara cream, containing the TLR7-ligand and potent immune activator Imiquimod (IMQ) (*see* **Note 1**), can induce and exacerbate psoriasis [3], van der Fits and colleagues recently developed a novel psoriasis model. Daily painting of Aldara/IMQ cream onto mouse skin triggers the development of inflamed scaly skin lesions closely resembling plaque-type psoriasis. In particular, Aldara/IMQ-induced dermatitis is mediated via the IL-23/IL-17 axis and only partially dependent on T cells [4]. The unique power of this rapid and convenient model lies in dissecting the early cellular and molecular events during psoriatic plaque formation. Using the Aldara/IMQ-model we and others recently discovered the critical role of innate lymphocytes, in particular γδ T cells [5, 6], and conventional DC [7] in the initiation of psoriasiform skin inflammation. In this chapter, we provide a detailed description of the induction and phenotype of Aldara/IMQ-mediated skin inflammation, and the analysis of DC and innate lymphocyte populations as well as intracellular cytokine production by flow cytometry following topical Aldara/IMQ treatment.

## 2 Materials

### 2.1 Induction of IMQ-Mediated Psoriasiform Skin Inflammation

1. 7–9-week-old, sex- and weight-matched mice (*see* **Notes 2–4**).
2. Shaving device.
3. Aldara cream containing 5 % IMQ.
4. Control vehicle cream.
5. Micrometer.
6. Small spatula.
7. Balance.

### 2.2 Immuno-histochemical Analysis of Aldara-Induced Dermatitis

1. Biopsy puncher to collect 3 mm back- and ear-skin samples.
2. Standard equipment to prepare 6 μm cross sections of the cryo-preserved skin, including TissueTek, liquid nitrogen, and cryostat.

### 2.3 Analysis of the Leukocyte Skin Infiltrate by Flow Cytometry

#### 2.3.1 Preparation of Skin Single-Cell Suspension

1. Standard laboratory equipment including cell culture dishes, 70-μm nylon cell strainers, and fluorescence-activated cell sorting (FACS) tubes.
2. RPMI 1640 Medium supplemented with 1 % penicillin-streptomycin and 25 mM HEPES.
3. Digestion medium: RPMI supplemented with 10 mM HEPES, 400 U/ml collagenase IV, 100 U/ml hyaluronidase, and 0.1 % DNAse.
4. 0.5 M EDTA.

#### 2.3.2 Flow Cytometry

1. FACS buffer consisting of PBS containing 2.6 mM $KH_2PO_4$, 26 mM $Na_2HPO_4$, 145 mM NaCl, final pH 7.2 supplemented with 2 % fetal calf serum and 0.02 % thimerosal.
2. 4 % Paraformaldehyde (PFA) in PBS as stock solution, diluted 1:2 in FACS buffer to a 2 % solution.
3. Perm/wash solution of 0.1 % saponin in FACS buffer (=0.025 g/10 ml).
4. Purified and unlabeled CD16/32 antibody (Fc-Block).
5. Fixable dead cell stain.
6. The specifics and source of monoclonal antibodies (mAbs) used for flow cytometry are provided in Tables 1 and 2.

**Table 1**
**mAbs used for FACS analysis of innate lymphocytes**

| Specificity | Clone | Species | Isotype | Supplier |
|---|---|---|---|---|
| CD3 | 17A2 | Rat | IgG2bκ | Biolegend |
| CD4 | RM4-5 | Rat | IgG | Biolegend |
| CD5 | 53-7.3 | Rat | IgG2aκ | Biolegend |
| CD11c | N418 | Arm. hamster | IgG | Biolegend |
| CD45 | 30-F11 | Rat | IgG2bκ | Biolegend |
| CD45R (B220) | RA3-682 | Rat | IgG2aκ | Biolegend |
| CD90 (Thy1) | 30-H12 | Rat | IgG2bκ | Biolegend |
| CD127 (IL-7Ra) | SB/199 | Rat | IgG2aλ | Biolegend |
| Sca-1 (Ly-6A/E) | D7 | Rat | IgG2aκ | Biolegend |
| Gr-1 (Ly-6C/G) | RB6-8C5 | Rat | IgG2bκ | Biolegend |
| TCRγδ | GL3 | Hamster | IgG2κ | Biolegend |
| TCR Vγ2 (Vγ4) | UC3-10A6 | Arm. hamster | IgG | Biolegend |
| TCR Vγ3 (Vγ5) | 536 | Syr. hamster | IgG | Biolegend |

**Table 2**
**mAbs used for FACS analysis of DC**

| Specificity | Clone | Species | Isotype | Supplier |
|---|---|---|---|---|
| CD11b | M1/70 | Rat | IgG2bκ | Biolegend |
| CD11c | N418 | Arm. hamster | IgG | Biolegend |
| CD45 | 30-F11 | Rat | IgG2bκ | Biolegend |
| CD64 | X54-5/7.1 | Rat | IgG1bκ | Biolegend |
| Langerin | 929F3.1 | Rat | IgG2a | Dendritics |
| Ly6-G | 1A8 | Rat | IgG2bκ | Biolegend |
| MHCII I-A/I-E | M5/114.15.2 | Rat | IgG2bκ | Biolegend |
| MMR6 | MR5D3 | Rat | IgG2aκ | Biolegend |

### 2.4 In Vivo Brefeldin A Treatment to Detect Intracellular Cytokines

1. 20 mg/ml Brefeldin A solution in DMSO, to be further diluted in PBS to a final concentration of 0.5 mg/ml for in vivo inoculation.
2. Reagents for preparation of a skin single-cell suspension and FACS staining (Subheading 2.3).
3. Standard equipment for intravenous injection of mice.

## 3 Methods

### 3.1 Aldara Model of Psoriasis-Like Skin Inflammation

#### 3.1.1 Mouse Preparation and Aldara Treatment

1. One day before starting the Aldara treatment a large area of the back of the animals is shaved thoroughly (*see* **Note 5**).
2. To induce skin inflammation leading to psoriasis-like plaque formation, the mice receive a daily topical dose of 62.5 mg of commercially available Aldara cream on their shaved backs and one or both ears for up to 6 consecutive days (*see* **Note 6**). This represents a daily dose of 3.125 mg of IMQ [4]. Control animals are treated similarly with vehicle cream. An easy way to apply the cream onto the mouse skin is by using a small spatula.

#### 3.1.2 Scoring of Psoriasiform Skin Inflammation

Severity of inflammation is indicated by ear swelling and thickening of the back skin, as well as erythema and scaling, which is assessed by scoring a defined set of parameters (Fig. 1 and [4]). Increase in skin thickness and ear swelling during the disease course can be monitored with a micrometer. To calculate the relative increase in skin thickness a normalized value is calculated, based on baseline measurement before start of the Aldara treatment (Fig. 1b). Skin redness and scaling of the back skin are scored with an objective scoring system on a scale from 0 to 4 (0, none; 1, slight; 2, moderate;

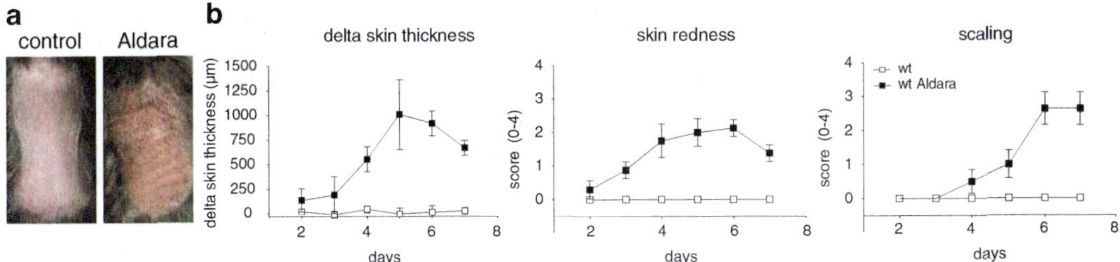


**Fig. 1** Aldara-induced skin inflammation in mice phenotypically resembles psoriasis. C57BL/6 mice were treated with Aldara for 6 consecutive days. (**a**) Pictures of representative mice on day 6. (**b**) Increase in back skin thickness, redness, and scaling during the course of disease

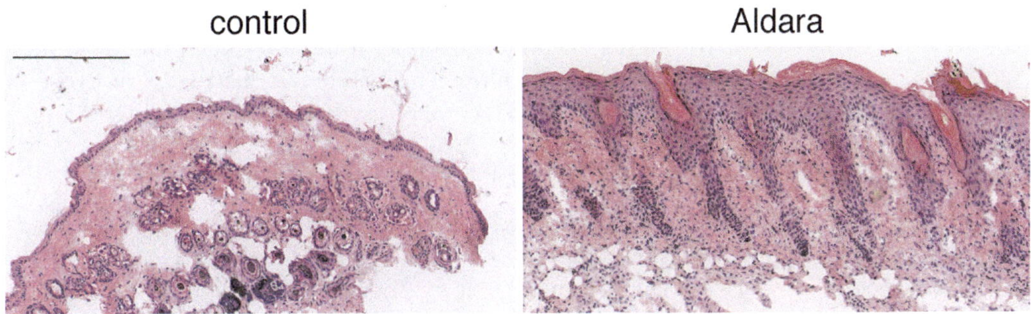


**Fig. 2** Psoriasiform epidermal thickening and rete ridges induced by Aldara application. Representative H&E-stained ear skin sections on day 6 of control and Aldara cream-treated mice. Magnification ×100, scale bar 100 μm

3, marked; 4, very marked) (Fig. 1b). For the level of redness a scoring table with red tints is used. This scoring system is based on the clinical Psoriasis Area and Severity Index (PASI), with the only exception that the skin thickness is measured while the size of the affected skin area is not taken into account [4].

### 3.2 Histology

1. Biopsies from back and ear skin (3 mm diameter) are immersed in TissueTek, snap-frozen in liquid nitrogen, and stored at −80 °C until use.
2. Six-micrometer cryosections of skin are cut using a cryostat.
3. Sections are stained with H&E following standard procedures (Fig. 2).

### 3.3 Flow Cytometry

To investigate cellular changes in the skin and the composition of the inflammatory cell infiltrate, skin samples are taken during the course of Aldara treatment and analyzed by flow cytometry. For this purpose, single-cell suspensions of back and/or ear skin are prepared and stained with appropriate panels of fluorescently labeled mAbs to discriminate different innate lymphocyte and dendritic cell populations (*see* Tables 1 and 2).

*3.3.1 Preparation of a Single-Cell Suspension*

1. Mice are sacrificed and ears and/or back skin are collected. Ears are split into dorsal and ventral halves with tweezers, starting at the cut edge. For the back skin samples the subdermal fat is removed in order to quench autofluorescence during FACS analysis. Tissues are kept on ice and cut into small pieces.
2. Following mechanical disruption the pieces of skin tissue are incubated in digestion medium (*see* Subheading 2.3.1 and **Note 7**) for 1.5 h at 37 °C in a shaking water bath or a thermoshaker (1,300 rpm).
3. Enzymatic digestion is stopped and cell clusters are disrupted by adding EDTA to the mix at a final concentration of 15 mM for an additional 5 min (*see* **Note 8**).
4. Single-cell suspensions are prepared by pushing the mixture through a 70-μm cell strainer using a syringe plunger to mash cells through the filter. The cells are washed 1× with PBS containing 2 mM EDTA (*see* **Note 9**) and spun down for 7 min at 400 × *g*.
5. Cells are resuspended in FACS buffer, transferred into FACS tubes, and counted to later determine absolute cell numbers.

*3.3.2 Staining Protocol for Flow Cytometric Analysis of Cell Surface Markers*

1. For surface staining, cell suspensions are divided over the number of stainings needed and preincubated on ice in 100 μl PBS containing fixable dead cell stain for at least 15 min.
2. Next, the cells are washed with PBS once, preincubated on ice in 50 μl FACS buffer containing Fc-Block (CD16/32) for at least 15 min, and labeled with cell surface Abs by adding 50 μl FACS buffer containing the appropriate mAbs (Ab cocktail depends on staining panel and cell type), followed by incubation at 4 °C for 30 min in the dark.
3. Following this incubation, the cells are washed and resuspended in FACS buffer (≥100 μl) and acquired immediately with a flow cytometer.

*3.3.3 Intracellular Staining Protocol for Flow Cytometry*

1. To detect intracellular molecules (e.g., cytokines), cell suspensions are fixed with 2 % PFA for 5 min.
2. The cells are washed with perm/wash once and stained with appropriate mAbs in 50 μl of perm/wash for 60 min at 4 °C in the dark.
3. After the staining cells are washed twice with perm/wash and once with FACS buffer.
4. Finally, cells are resuspended in FACS buffer and acquired within a week.

*3.3.4 Analysis of Skin Leukocyte Subsets by Flow Cytometry*

A good starting point of every FACS analysis is doublet exclusion, because doublets of DC and T cells will be fluorescent for markers of both cell types and therefore generate noise and confusion during

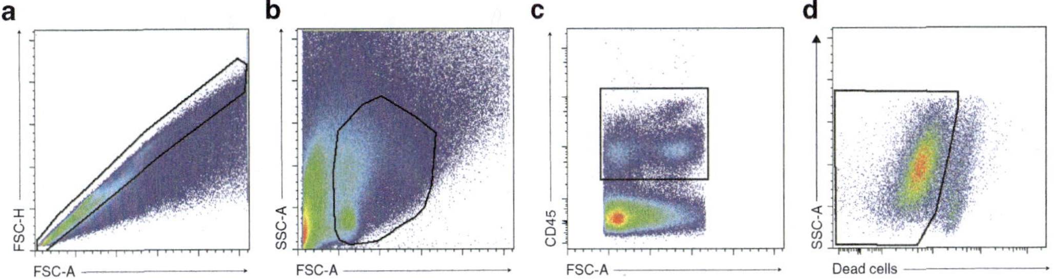


**Fig. 3** Gating strategy for efficient analysis of leukocytes in the skin. (**a**) Doublet discrimination. (**b**) Rough pre-gating on leukocytes. (**c**) Identification of leukocytes based on CD45 staining. (**d**) Live-cell gate

the subsequent gating procedure. Doublet discrimination is a process whereby the area forward scatter (FSC) (FSC-A) of the fluorescence light pulse is plotted against the height (FSC-H). Doublets will have greater pulse width than single cells, as they take longer to pass through the laser beam, and therefore can be excluded from the analysis by gating on the events positioned on a diagonal of FSC-A and FSC-H (Fig. 3a). In the next step, to exclude debris and the majority of dead cells, a rough leukocyte gate using FSC and side scatter (SSC) should be made. The easiest way to do so is to copy a leukocyte gate from the same experiment obtained for a secondary lymphoid organ such as a lymph node or a spleen, where drawing this gate is a lot more straightforward (Fig. 3b). To ensure that only leukocytes are included in the analysis the cells are next gated on $CD45^+$, which is ubiquitously expressed on leukocytes (Fig. 3c and *see* **Note 10**). Dead cells are highly autofluorescent and tend to bind antibodies unspecifically. To exclude these cells from the subsequent analysis fixable dead cell stain, which reacts with cellular proteins (amines), is used. The dye can permeate damaged membranes and stain both the interior and exterior amines resulting in intense staining. As the dye cannot penetrate the cell membrane of viable cells only surface proteins are labeled leading to a weak staining of live cells (Fig. 3d). The above gating strategy is highly recommended to achieve easy and intuitive analysis of the immune cells in the skin.

#### 3.3.5 FACS Analysis of γδ T Cells

γδ T cells are generally subdivided into subsets according to Vγ chain usage. However, two nomenclatures assigning numbers to Vγ chains appeared at the same time with one being preferentially used by antibody vendors [8] and the other more commonly found in research articles [9]. For clarification, the corresponding nomenclatures for Vγ chains used for the identification of γδ T cells in the skin are summarized in Table 3. From this point onwards Heilig and Tonegawa nomenclature will be used. In the steady state, γδ T cells in murine skin are predominantly $V\gamma5^+$ cells residing in the

**Table 3**
**γδ T cell nomenclature**

| Heilig and Tonegawa [9] | Garman [8] |
|---|---|
| Vγ1 | Vγ1.1 |
| Vγ2 | Vγ1.2 |
| Vγ3 | Vγ1.3 |
| Vγ4 | Vγ2 |
| Vγ5 | Vγ3 |
| Vγ6 | Vγ4 |
| Vγ7 | Vγ5 |

epidermis, called dendritic epidermal T cells (DETC) [10]. Dermal resident γδ T cells primarily express the Vγ4 chain [11, 12]. γδ T cells are distinct from B and αβ T cells in that they combine conventional adaptive features (inherent in their T cell receptors (TCR) and pleiotropic effector functions) with rapid, innate-like responses that can place them in the initiation phase of immune reactions (reviewed in [13]).

γδ T cells are a lot less studied than the conventional αβ T cells and there are no specific markers known apart from their γδ TCR. Due to a strict ratio of two CD3e molecules to a single δ chain within the γδ TCR complex, γδ T cells will appear on the diagonal when those two stainings are analyzed together (Fig. 4a). Gate I represents γδ T cells, while Gate II comprises all other T cells present in the skin. Two populations are clearly visible within Gate I. The higher population represents nearly exclusively epidermal DETC. This subset of γδ T cells exhibits a dendritic morphology, resulting in a greater surface area and hence higher expression levels of TCR γδ per cell as compared to other γδ T cells, which results in a more intense staining. The lower population of $CD3^{+}TCR\gamma\delta^{+}$ represents the dermal subsets of γδ T cells. As can be seen in Fig. 4b, a large proportion of these cells are $V\gamma4^{+}$. Finally, Fig. 4c confirms that the upper population of $CD3^{+}TCR\gamma\delta^{+}$ cells are indeed $V\gamma5^{+}$ DETC. As depicted in the bottom part of Fig. 4, upon Aldara treatment the percentage of DETC is significantly reduced, but the absolute numbers remain relatively constant, while $V\gamma4^{+}$ cells drastically increase. In the context of Aldara-driven psoriasis-like inflammation $V\gamma4^{+}$ γδ T cells are the main source of IL-17A, IL-17F, and IL-22. These cytokines are the main drivers of the inflammation observed during Aldara treatment [5, 6].

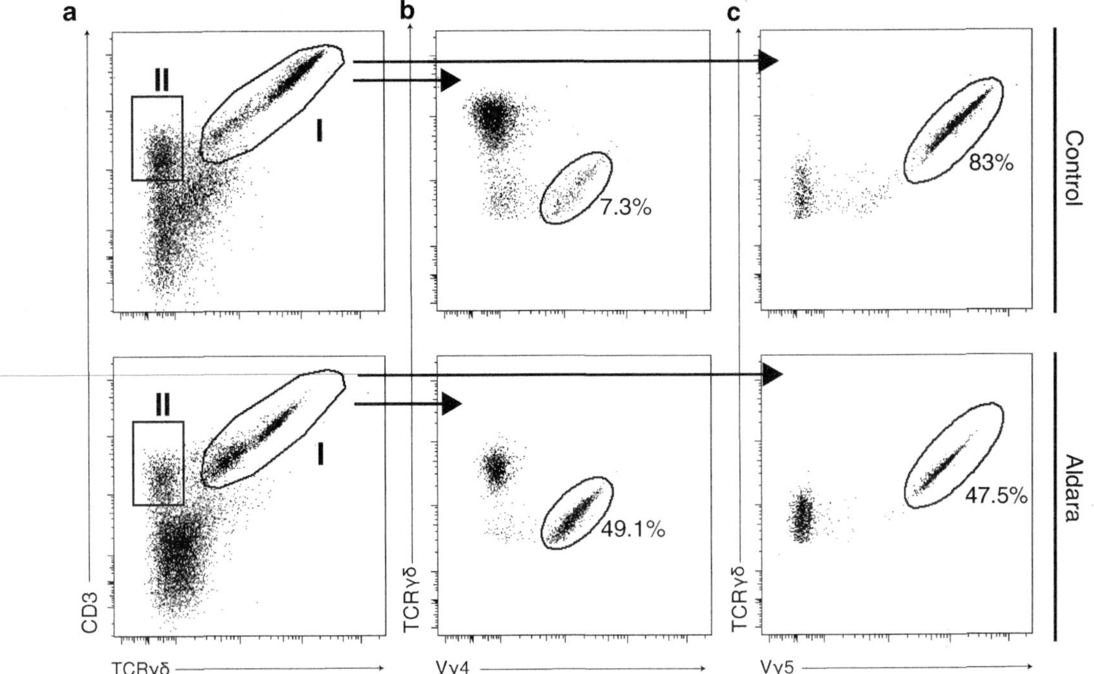


**Fig. 4** Gating strategy to dissect γδ T cell subsets in the skin. (**a**) Gating on γδ (I) and other T cells (II) in the skin. (**b**) The lower population of $CD3^{+}TCR\gamma\delta^{+}$ cells represents dermal γδ T cell subsets, which include $V\gamma4^{+}$ cells. (**c**) The higher population are $V\gamma5^{+}$ DETCs

#### 3.3.6 FACS Analysis of Innate Lymphoid Cells (ILC)

ILC are a family of developmentally related cells involved in immunity as well as tissue development and remodeling. These cells have been recently identified for their cytokine production patterns, which are very similar to those of T helper cell subsets (reviewed in [14]). Recent findings implicate ILC to have important effector functions during the early stages of immune responses against microorganisms, tissue repair, and inflammatory diseases. However, due to the fact that they are very rare cells (even more so than γδ T cells) and that no specific markers are known, gating for ILC is complex and cumbersome.

As ILC are lineage-negative cells the easiest way to identify them is by setting up a "dump" channel with lineage markers (CD11c, Gr-1, B220, and CD5). When the dump channel is displayed against CD3 only a very small population of cells in the skin is negative for all lineage markers and includes ILC (Fig. 5a). On the other hand, these cells are positive for Sca-1 and Thy-1 (Fig. 5b), as well as IL-7Rα (Fig. 5c) [15]. Extreme caution and very conservative gating is recommended for these cells as it is still very hard to identify ILC by means of FACS without the aid of transgenic mice (*see* **Note 11**). In the absence of γδ T cells ILC provide an alternative source of IL-22 in the Aldara skin inflammation model, which explains the residual inflammation observed in *Tcrd*$^{-/-}$ and *Rag1*$^{-/-}$ mice [6].

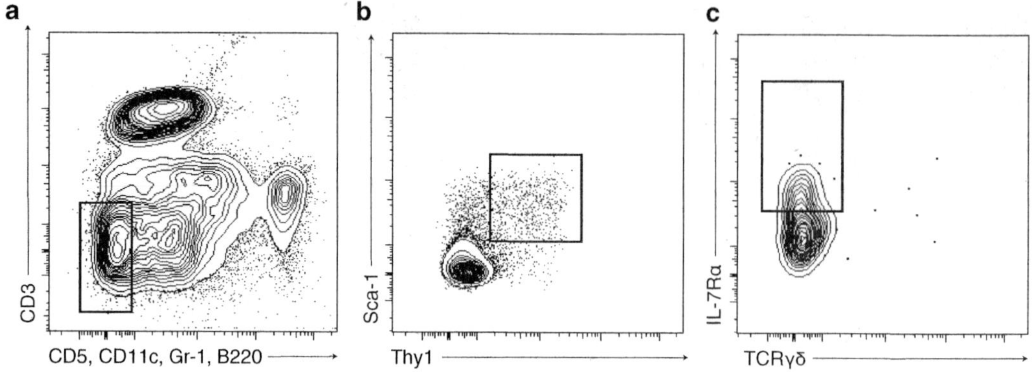


**Fig. 5** Gating strategy for identification of ILCs in the skin. (**a**) Gating on ILCs by excluding lineage-positive cells. (**b**, **c**) ILCs are positive for Sca-1, Thy1, and IL-7Rα

**Table 4**
**Phenotype of skin DC subsets**

| Skin DC subset | Phenotype | | | | |
|---|---|---|---|---|---|
| *Epidermis* | | | | | |
| LC | **Langerin$^+$** | CD11b$^{int}$ | CD103$^{neg}$ | **EpCam$^{++}$** | **CD24$^+$** |
| *Dermis* | | | | | |
| LC in transit | **Langerin$^+$** | CD11b$^{int}$ | CD103$^{neg}$ | **EpCam$^{++}$** | **CD24$^+$** |
| CD11b$^+$Langerin$^{neg}$ dDC | Langerin$^{neg}$ | **CD11b$^{high}$** | CD103$^{neg}$ | EpCam$^{neg}$ | CD24$^{neg}$ |
| CD11b$^{neg}$Langerin$^{neg}$ dDC | Langerin$^{neg}$ | CD11b$^{neg/lo}$ | CD103$^{neg}$ | EpCam$^{neg}$ | CD24$^{neg}$ |
| Langerin$^+$CD103$^{neg}$ dDC | **Langerin$^+$** | CD11b$^{lo}$ | CD103$^{neg}$ | EpCam$^{neg/lo}$ | **CD24$^+$** |
| Langerin$^+$CD103$^+$ dDC | **Langerin$^+$** | CD11b$^{lo}$ | **CD103$^+$** | EpCam$^{neg}$ | **CD24$^+$** |
| CD11b$^+$ moDC[a] | Langerin$^{neg}$ | **CD11b$^+$** | CD103$^{neg}$ | EpCam$^{neg}$ | CD24$^{neg}$ |

Bold text indicates positive markers
*dDC* dermal DC
[a]Inflammatory moDC are characterized by the expression of CD64 [19, 20]. Adapted from [16]

*3.3.7 FACS Analysis of Dendritic Cells*

In steady state skin there are two major DC populations: Langerin$^+$ epidermal Langerhans cells (LC) and dermal DC. The latter can be further subdivided into a small subset of Langerin$^+$ dermal DC that differ from LC by the expression of CD103 and EpCam, and Langerin$^{neg}$ dermal DC that are CD103$^{+/neg}$ (Table 4 and [16]).

To study skin DC populations during Aldara-induced inflammation, resident and infiltrating leukocytes are identified by gating on singlets and live CD45$^+$ cells as illustrated in Fig. 3. DC are then identified by expression of MHCII$^+$ and CD11c$^+$ (Fig. 6a) and can be further divided into Langerin$^+$ and CD11b$^+$ subpopulations

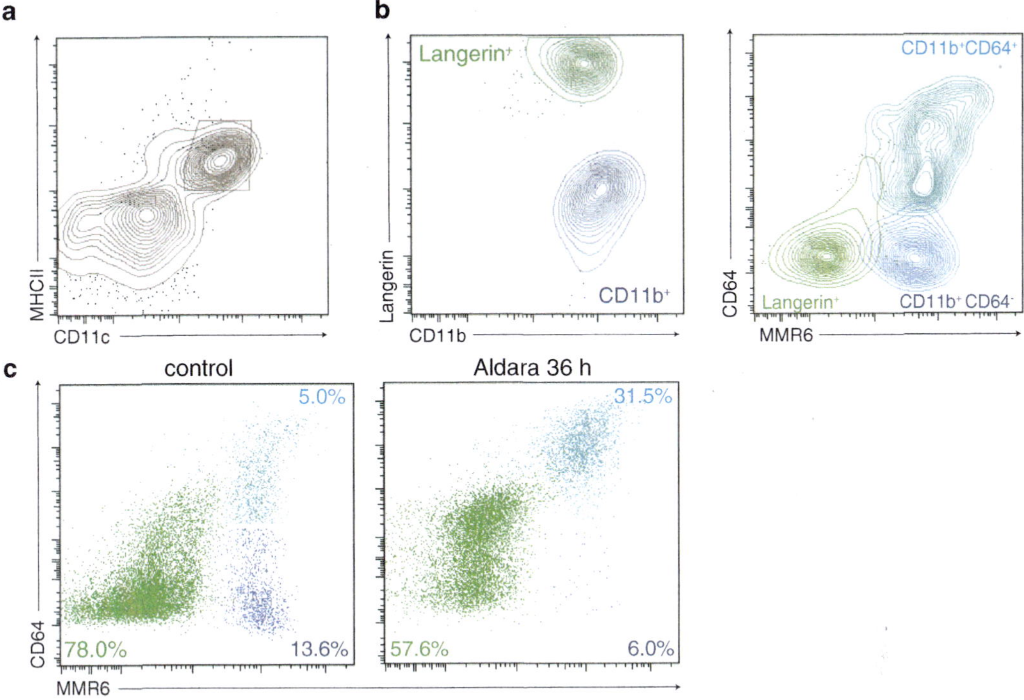


**Fig. 6** Gating strategy to discriminate different skin DC subsets. (**a**) Gating on MHCII+CD11c+ DC. (**b**, **c**) Identification of Langerin+, CD11b+, and monocyte-derived CD64+MMR6+ inflammatory DC populations

[16–18] (Fig. 6b and *see* **Note 12**). In a whole skin cell preparation Langerin+ DC comprise epidermal LC and dermal Langerin+ DC, which can be dissected by differential expression of CD103 and EpCam (Table 3). As shown in Fig. 6b, infiltrating monocyte-derived DC (moDC) are distinguished from dermal resident CD11b+ DC by expression of the high-affinity IgG receptor FcγR1 (CD64) [19, 20]. The macrophage mannose receptor (MMR)6 (CD206) is expressed at high levels by macrophages and moDC, as well as at lower levels by other DC subsets, including Langerhans cells [21, 22]. MMR6 should be detected by intracellular FACS staining, as collagen fragments, which are inevitably generated during collagenase digestion, bind to MMR6 and cause its internalization following binding [23].

Topical application of Aldara cream leads to migration of skin DC, including LC to the draining lymph nodes for the activation of adaptive T cell responses [24]. At the same time, monocytes are recruited to the site of inflammation and differentiate into DC in situ [25]. Newly formed moDC may play essential roles inducing both innate and adaptive immune reactions. Figure 6c depicts the accumulation of CD64+CD11b+ moDC during Aldara-driven skin inflammation.

### 3.4 In Vivo Brefeldin A Treatment to Detect Intracellular Cytokines

To unravel the cell type-specific contribution to regulatory networks during Aldara-induced psoriatic plaque formation, detection of in vivo cytokine production in response to Aldara cream can be very useful. To this aim, we adapted a previously described protocol using inoculation of brefeldin A in vivo [26] (*see* **Note 13**). Our data demonstrated that IL-23, which drives the activation of γδ T cells and ILC, is exclusively produced by a Langerin$^{neg}$ skin DC subset [7].

1. Mice are injected intravenously with 0.25 mg brefeldin A (*see* **Notes 14–16**) prior to a single topical application of Aldara cream onto both ears. Control animals are brefeldin A-injected and painted with vehicle cream.
2. 12 h after treatment (*see* **Note 17**), whole-ear skin cell suspensions are prepared and analyzed for cell surface markers and intracellular cytokines by flow cytometry as described above (*see* Subheading 3.3).

## 4 Notes

1. The approximate composition of Aldara cream is published [27] and it contains other ingredients than IMQ that can lead to activation of the inflammasome, keratinocyte death, and IL-1 release [28]. We however observed that MyD88 knockout mice are completely resistant to Aldara-mediated skin inflammation indicating that TLR and IL-1 signaling are critical for psoriatic plaque development in this model [7].
2. Aldara-mediated skin inflammation can in principle be induced in every inbred mouse strain, but the degree of skin inflammation might vary. From our own experience, the inflammation and development of psoriatic plaques are more pronounced and obvious in Balb/c animals [4]. Due to the predominant background of transgenic and/or knockout mice, we routinely elicit and analyze Aldara-induced skin inflammation in C57BL/6 mice (Fig. 1a).
3. The reaction and development of the inflammatory skin phenotype are exacerbated in female as compared to male mice, probably due to differences in skin thickness and weight, but also sex-specific strength of TLR7 responses [29, 30]. Therefore, we recommend to preferentially use female animals and not to mix sexes in experimental groups.
4. Due to slow hair growth in mice between weeks 7 and 9 after birth, it is desirable to apply Aldara onto the back skin during this age. In case the animals are older, ear treatment alone can be used to induce psoriatic plaque formation with a slightly delayed peak of inflammation (days 7–8).

5. Alternatively to shaving and, in particular, to facilitate detection of intricate phenotypes, hair depilation cream can be applied onto the mouse back. Moreover, differential shaving between individual mice can cause different retention times of Aldara on the skin, leading to a greater variation in the magnitude of the inflammatory phenotype.
6. To prevent excessive weight loss (greater than 10 % of body weight), in particular in C57BL/6 mice, animals can be injected with 250 μl PBS on days 2 and/or 3 of Aldara treatment.
7. Collagenases IV and D purchased from Sigma or Worthington are used with comparable efficiency in both our laboratories to prepare cutaneous single-cell suspensions.
8. To prevent "over-digestion" we strongly recommend adding EDTA at a final concentration of 15 mM to the digestion medium.
9. Buffers for FACS staining and washing steps should contain 2 mM EDTA to reduce the number of duplexes (i.e., DC:T cell aggregates) in the cell suspensions.
10. In case the exact location of leukocytes after doublet exclusion is difficult to determine in the FSC-A versus SSC-A plot, a rough gate can be set on $CD45^+$ cells. This will considerably reduce the number of events not representing leukocytes.
11. To ensure proper gating on ILC we recommend using "RORγt-fate map mice" (Rorc(γt)-$Cre^{Tg}$;$Rosa26R^{Eyfp/+}$) [31]. In this transgenic mouse strain every ILC will be $CD3^{neg}$ and $EYFP^+$.
12. If necessary, intracellular staining for Langerin in DC subsets can be replaced with extracellular detection of CD24, as expression of these markers overlaps on the corresponding DC subsets (Table 4 and [16]).
13. Depending on the cellular source of the cytokine to be analyzed the appropriate timing is of vital importance. If the cytokine-producing cell type is directly activated by Aldara/IMQ (e.g., like DC are direct targets of IMQ) brefeldin A should be injected immediately prior to the treatment. In case the cytokine secretion to be analyzed represents a secondary response (like for T cells) a considerable amount of time should be given between Aldara treatment and brefeldin A injection; otherwise the response might be lost due to blocking of cytokine secretion by primary responding cells like DC.
14. The recommended amount of 0.25 mg brefeldin A should be injected in the indicated volume of 500 μl. This will ensure a uniform distribution of brefeldin A within the body. Following injection the heart rate will temporarily increase, but should go back to normal after 1–2 min.

15. Due to this rather high injection volume it is recommended to warm up the brefeldin A solution to body temperature to prevent the tail vein from collapsing. In addition, brefeldin A should be injected slowly to reduce discomfort for the animals.
16. Brefeldin A can also be solubilized in ethanol instead of DMSO. However, we *do not* recommend this, since the rather high dosage of ethanol causes major discomfort for the animals and does interfere with immune responses.
17. For ethical reasons mice *must not* be treated for more than 12 h with brefeldin A, as it blocks secretion of soluble mediators from all cells of the body.

## References


1. Perera GK, Di Meglio P, Nestle FO (2012) Psoriasis. Annu Rev Pathol Mech Dis 7:385–422
2. Schön MP (2008) Animal models of psoriasis: a critical appraisal. Exp Dermatol 17:703–712
3. Gilliet M, Conrad C, Geiges M et al (2004) Psoriasis triggered by toll-like receptor 7 agonist imiquimod in the presence of dermal plasmacytoid dendritic cell precursors. Arch Dermatol 140:1490–1495
4. van der Fits L, Mourits S, Voerman JSA et al (2009) Imiquimod-induced psoriasis-like skin inflammation in mice is mediated via the IL-23/IL-17 Axis. J Immunol 182:5836–5845
5. Cai Y, Shen X, Ding C et al (2011) Pivotal role of dermal IL-17-producing γt T cells in skin inflammation. Immunity 35:596–610
6. Pantelyushin S, Haak S, Ingold B et al (2012) Rorγt+innate lymphocytes and γδ T cells initiate psoriasiform plaque formation in mice. J Clin Invest 122:2252–2256
7. Wohn C, Ober-Blöbaum JL, Haak S et al (2013) Langerin$^{neg}$ conventional dendritic cells produce IL-23 to drive psoriatic plaque formation in mice. Proc Natl Acad Sci U S A 110(26): 10723–10728
8. Garman RD, Doherty PJ, Raulet DH (1986) Diversity, rearrangement, and expression of murine T cell gamma genes. Cell 45:733–742
9. Heilig JS, Tonegawa S (1986) Diversity of murine gamma genes and expression in fetal and adult T lymphocytes. Nature 322:836–840
10. Havran WL, Grell S, Duwe G et al (1989) Limited diversity of T-cell receptor gamma-chain expression of murine Thy-1+ dendritic epidermal cells revealed by V gamma 3-specific monoclonal antibody. Proc Natl Acad Sci U S A 86:4185–4189
11. Gray EE, Suzuki K, Cyster JG (2011) Cutting edge: identification of a motile IL-17-producing T cell population in the dermis. J Immunol 186:6091–6095
12. Sumaria N, Roediger B, Ng LG et al (2011) Cutaneous immunosurveillance by self-renewing dermal T cells. J Exp Med 208:505–518
13. Vantourout P, Hayday A (2013) Six-of-the-best: unique contributions of γδ T cells to immunology. Nat Rev Immunol 13:88–100
14. Bernink J, Mjösberg J, Spits H (2013) Th1- and Th2-like subsets of innate lymphoid cells. Immunol Rev 252:133–138
15. Buonocore S, Ahern PP, Uhlig HH et al (2010) Innate lymphoid cells drive interleukin-23-dependent innate intestinal pathology. Nature 464:1371–1375
16. Henri S, Poulin LF, Tamoutounour S et al (2010) CD207+ CD103+ dermal dendritic cells cross-present keratinocyte-derived antigens irrespective of the presence of Langerhans cells. J Exp Med 207:189–206
17. Clausen BE, Kel JM (2010) Langerhans cells: critical regulators of skin immunity? Immunol Cell Biol 88:351–360
18. Romani N, Clausen BE, Stoitzner P (2010) Langerhans cells and more: langerin-expressing dendritic cell subsets in the skin. Immunol Rev 234:120–141
19. Langlet C, Tamoutounour S, Henri S et al (2012) CD64 expression distinguishes monocyte-derived and conventional dendritic cells and reveals their distinct role during intramuscular Immunization. J Immunol 188: 1751–1760
20. Plantinga M, Guilliams M, Vanheerswynghels M et al (2013) Conventional and monocyte-derived CD11b+dendritic cells initiate and maintain T helper 2 cell-mediated immunity to house dust mite allergen. Immunity 38:322–335
21. Wollenberg A, Mommaas M, Oppel T et al (2002) Expression and function of the mannose

receptor CD206 on epidermal dendritic cells in inflammatory skin diseases. J Invest Dermatol 118:327–334

22. Cheong C, Matos I, Choi J-H et al (2010) Microbial stimulation fully differentiates monocytes to DC-SIGN/CD209+ dendritic cells for immune T cell areas. Cell 143: 416–429
23. Burgdorf S, Schuette V, Semmling V et al (2010) Steady state cross-presentation of OVA is mannose receptor-dependent but inhibitable by collagen fragments. Proc Natl Acad Sci U S A 107:E48–E49
24. Suzuki H, Wang B, Shivji GM et al (2000) Imiquimod, a topical immune response modifier, induces migration of Langerhans cells. J Invest Dermatol 114:135–141
25. Domínguez P, Ardavín C (2010) Differentiation and function of mouse monocyte-derived dendritic cells in steady state and inflammation. Immunol Rev 234(90–104):1–15
26. Liu F, Whitton JL (2005) Cutting edge: re-evaluating the in vivo cytokine responses of CD8+ T cells during primary and secondary viral infections. J Immunol 174:5936–5940
27. Heib V, Becker M, Warger T et al (2007) Mast cells are crucial for early inflammation, migration of Langerhans cells, and CTL responses following topical application of TLR7 ligand in mice. Blood 110:946–953
28. Walter A, Schäfer M, Cecconi V et al (2013) Aldara activates TLR7-independent immune defence. Nat Commun 4:1560
29. Berghöfer B, Frommer T, Haley G et al (2006) TLR7 ligands induce higher IFN-alpha production in females. J Immunol 177: 2088–2096
30. Karnam G, Rygiel TP, Raaben M et al (2012) CD200 receptor controls sex-specific TLR7 responses to viral infection. PLoS Pathog 8:e1002710
31. Vonarbourg C, Mortha A, Bui VL et al (2010) Regulated expression of nuclear receptor RORγt confers distinct functional fates to NK cell receptor-expressing RORγt+innate lymphocytes. Immunity 33:736–751

# Chapter 17

# Induction of Passive EAE Using Myelin-Reactive CD4+ T Cells

**Rhoanne C. McPherson, Helen E. Cambrook, Richard A. O'Connor, and Stephen M. Anderton**

## Abstract

Experimental autoimmune encephalomyelitis (EAE) is an autoimmune disease of the central nervous system (CNS) often used as a model for the early inflammatory stages of multiple sclerosis and also as a model of organ-specific autoimmune disease.

This protocol describes the induction of passive EAE in mice, either using T cells isolated from mice primed with myelin antigens, or through the use of naïve TCR transgenic T cells activated in vitro in the presence of myelin-derived antigens.

**Key words** Experimental autoimmune encephalomyelitis, T cells, CNS, Autoimmune disease, Cytokines

## 1 Introduction

In active EAE, the induction of disease relies upon initiation of a peripheral immune response following immunization with myelin antigens in adjuvant. Subsequently, activated myelin-reactive CD4+ T cells migrate into the CNS and orchestrate immune-mediated damage to the myelin sheath surrounding neurons. Passive EAE offers an alternative approach using the transfer of pre-activated myelin-reactive CD4+ T cells into naïve host mice, without the requirement for immunization of the hosts. This adoptive transfer model offers many advantages over the active induction of EAE. Most notably, the lack of immunization in the host circumvents any nonspecific effects caused by the adjuvant, and avoids the establishment of an antigen depot within the periphery of the mice. With the use of congenic markers, pathogenic donor T cells can be traced and their specific role in disease progression investigated. The use of this approach provided definitive evidence that EAE is a CD4+ T cell-mediated disease [1, 2].

Ari Waisman and Burkhard Becher (eds.), *T-Helper Cells: Methods and Protocols*, Methods in Molecular Biology, vol. 1193, DOI 10.1007/978-1-4939-1212-4_17, © Springer Science+Business Media New York 2014

The use of mice with a defined genetic alteration (either as the source of donor T cells or as host mice) also allows for exploration of the importance of the gene in question to the disease process, when expressed specifically within, or everywhere but, the pathogenic T cell population. This serves as a simple and quick alternative to the generation of mice with T cell-specific genetic alterations, although equivalent conclusions cannot always be drawn from these two approaches.

There are two main strategies for inducing passive EAE:

(a) The transfer of T cells activated in vivo by immunization of wild type (WT) mice: the pathogenicity of these T cells is most often ensured by a brief in vitro restimulation with the relevant myelin autoantigen.

(b) The isolation of naïve T cells from myelin-responsive TCR transgenic mice, followed by their primary TCR activation in vitro (either with antigen or with anti-CD3) and their transfer into non-transgenic host mice.

The myelin autoantigen used for the activation of myelin-reactive T cells is determined by the strain of the WT mice and, where used, the TCR transgenic mice (Table 1), and most often includes the use of encephalitogenic peptides from either myelin basic protein (MBP), myelin oligodendrocyte glycoprotein (MOG) or proteolipid protein (PLP).

Various polarization protocols have been employed during the in vitro activation/reactivation stage to produce encephalitogenic T cells. These include protocols that polarize cells to Th1, Th17, Th9, and GM-CSF-producing phenotypes [3–5]. Although these

**Table 1**
**Mouse strains, MHC II-restricted myelin epitopes, and TCR transgenic mice used for EAE**

| Antigen | Peptide epitope | Mouse strain | TCR transgenic |
|---|---|---|---|
| MBP | Ac1–9 | PL/J | T/R+ [21] |
| | | | Tg4 [12] |
| | Ac1–11 | B10.PL [22] | H-2$^u$ αβ [23] |
| | Ac1–16 | B10.PL | MBP Tg+ [24] |
| | 80–100 and variants thereof | SJL/J [25] | |
| PLP | 139–151 | SJL/J [26] | 5B6 [27] |
| | 178–191 | SJL/J [28] | |
| | 56–70 | Biozzi/ABH [29] | |
| MOG | 8–21 | Biozzi/ABH [30] | |
| | 35–55 | C57BL/6 [31] | 2D2 [32] |
| | | Biozzi/ABH [30] | |
| | | PL/J [33]_ENREF_33 | [30] |
| | 92–106 | SJL | |

terms are used widely, it is our view that it is safest to restrict their use to protocols in which naïve TCR transgenic cells receive primary stimulation (in vitro) in a controlled manner. This produces the "cleanest" Th cell subsets. In vivo activation following immunization, although more physiological, is less controlled and usually promotes mixed T cell populations (even including those producing Th2-cytokines). In light of this, and to be consistent with those whose work we cite [6, 7], in this chapter we therefore refer to "IL-12-conditioned", or "IL-23-conditioned" populations from immunized WT mice. Note that, although IL-12 and IL-23 are the key ingredients to these two conditions, other cytokines may be added, or inhibited, during these cultures. Irrespective of the polarization or conditioning protocol employed, pathogenicity appears to be dictated by the ability of the effector T cells to produce GM-CSF rather than their predominant Th phenotype [5]. Here we describe several protocols that produce encephalitogenic T cells from both WT and TCR transgenic mice.

## 2 Materials

### 2.1 Generation of Pathogenic T Cells and the Induction of EAE

1. Complete Freund's adjuvant (CFA): containing 1 mg/ml heat-killed *Mycobacterium tuberculosis* H37Ra (*M. tuberculosis*) (Sigma-Aldrich, Poole, UK) (*see* **Note 1**).
2. Myelin-derived peptides: MOG (35–55) (MEVGWYRSPFS RVVHLYRNNGK) or acetylated MBP Ac1–9 (Ac-ASQK RPSQR) (Cambridge Research Biochemicals, Teesside, UK) (*see* **Note 2**).
3. Pertussis toxin (PTx) (Health Protection Agency, Dorset, UK).
4. Wash buffer: RPMI 1640 medium containing 25 mM Hepes.
5. RPMI-10 %: wash buffer, supplemented with 2 mM L-Glutamine, 100 U/ml Penicillin, 100 μg/ml Streptomycin, 50 μM 2-mercaptoethanol, and 10 % heat-inactivated fetal calf serum.
6. Sterile gauze (150 μM).
7. 15 ml and 50 ml Falcon conical centrifuge tubes.
8. 6-well flat bottom cell culture plates, or 75 $cm^2$ vented (T75) cell culture flasks.
9. RBC lysis buffer: containing 8.3 g/L ammonium chloride in 0.01 M Tris–HCl.
10. Trypan blue.
11. Sterile PBS (without $Mg^{2+}$ or $Ca^{2+}$).
12. Antibodies for cell culture: anti-CD3 and anti-CD28 (eBioscience, Hatfield, UK), anti-IFNγ (XMG1.2), anti-IL-12 (C17.8), and anti-IL-4 (A11B11) (all Bio X cell, USA).

13. Mouse recombinant cytokines; rIL-2, rIL-12, rIL-18, rTGF-β, rIL-23, rIL-4, rIL-1α (all R&D Systems, UK), rIL-6 (Miltenyi Biotec, Germany).
14. Ficoll-Paque PLUS (density of 1.007 g/ml).
15. Percoll gradient: 30 and 70 % Percoll (density of 1.135 g/ml) solutions diluted in wash buffer.
16. Digestion buffer: 2.5 mg/ml Collagenase IV (Lorne laboratories, UK) and 1 mg/ml deoxyribonuclease (DNase).
17. All mice used should be 6–10 weeks of age.

### 2.2 Phenotypic Analysis of T Cells

1. Phorbol myristate acetate (PMA) and ionomycin, Brefeldin A (eBioscience).
2. Fix/perm buffers: BD Cytofix/Cytoperm and Perm/Wash buffer (BD Pharmingen), Foxp3 Fixation/Permeabilization buffer and permeabilization buffer (eBioscience).
3. FACS buffer: PBS, 2 % Fetal calf serum (Sigma), 0.01 % $NaN_3$ (Sigma).
4. Antibodies and stains for flow cytometry: Fixable Viability Dye eFluor 780, anti-CD4 AlexaFluor 700, anti-GM-CSF PE (both BD), anti-T-bet PerCP-Cy5.5, anti-RORγt PE, anti-IFN-γ FITC, anti-TNF-α eFluor 450, and anti-IL-17 PerCP-Cy5.5 (all eBioscience). For all intracellular antigens appropriate isotype controls were used.
5. Ready-SET-Go! ELISA sets for detection of mouse IFNγ, IL-17A, GM-CSF, or TNFα (eBioscience).

## 3 Methods

### 3.1 Polyclonal Passive EAE

This section outlines the generation of pathogenic myelin-reactive CD4+ T cells from primed susceptible mouse strains. C57BL/6 (H-$2^b$) mice are used widely due to the number of genetically altered lines on this background. However, the same general protocols can be used for other strains with alternative peptides or CNS antigens (Table 1).

#### 3.1.1 Immunization of Donor Mice

Immunize donor mice with 100 μg of MOG (35–55) emulsified in CFA containing 200 μg of *M. tuberculosis*. Mice receive a total volume of 100 μl, injected subcutaneously (s.c.); 50 μl into each hind leg (*see* **Note 3**). Adapted from O'Connor et al. [8].

#### 3.1.2 Passive EAE Using IL-12-Conditioned Cells (Adapted from Ito et al. [9])

1. After 7–10 days harvest draining lymph nodes and spleen as required, keep tissues in wash buffer on ice until processed.
2. Create a single cell suspension in wash buffer by pushing cells through 150 μM sterile gauze or equivalent cell strainer.

3. To pellet/wash cells centrifuge at $350 \times g$ for 5 min (as for all subsequent wash steps unless otherwise stated).
4. If taking spleen, lyse red blood cells at room temperature for 2 min using 2 ml RBC lysis buffer per spleen, and wash once in wash buffer.
5. Resuspend cells in wash buffer and count viable cells using trypan blue exclusion.
6. Culture cells at $4 \times 10^6$/ml in RPMI-10 % containing 10 μg/ml MOG (35–55), 10 U/ml rIL-2, 25 ng/ml rIL-12, and 25 ng/ml rIL-18 in 6-well plates (4–6 ml per well) at 37 °C, 5 % $CO_2$ in a humidified atmosphere (*see* **Note 4**).
7. After 48 h split the cells and increase the concentration of IL-2 to 20 U/ml for the final 24 h
8. At the end of culture, keep an aliquot of cells and an aliquot of culture supernatant to analyze cytokine production by flow cytometry and ELISA respectively (Subheading 3.4)
9. Harvest the activated lymphocytes by gently washing off the plate with PBS and place in a 50 ml falcon tube
10. Wash cells three times in sterile PBS and count viable blasting (enlarged) cells using trypan blue exclusion
11. Inject $4 \times 10^6$ blasts in a total volume of 200 μl PBS intravenously (i.v.) into C57BL/6 hosts (*see* **Notes 5** and **6**)
12. In addition, inject 200 ng PTx in 500 μl PBS i.p. on the same day as cell transfer

#### *3.1.3 Passive EAE Using IL-23-Conditioned Cells (Adapted from Kroenke et al. [10])*

1. After 7–10 days harvest draining lymph nodes and spleen as required, and create a single cell suspension (Subheading 3.1.2, **steps 2–5**)
2. Culture cells at $4 \times 10^6$/ml in RPMI-10 % containing 50 μg/ml MOG (35–55), 8 ng/ml rIL-23, 10 ng/ml rIL-1α, 10 μg/ml anti-IL-4, and 10 μg/ml anti-IFNγ
3. Culture for 96 h in 30 ml volumes in T75 flasks at 37 °C, 5 % $CO_2$ in a humidified atmosphere (*see* **Note** 7)
4. At the end of culture, keep an aliquot of cells and an aliquot of culture supernatant to analyze cytokine production by flow cytometry and ELISA respectively (Subheading 3.4)
5. Harvest activated lymphocytes, and purify live cells by separation over a Ficoll gradient (as per manufacturer's instructions)
6. Wash cells and inject $4 \times 10^6$ blasts per host (Subheading 3.1.2, **steps 10–12**). No PTx is required with this protocol (*see* **Note 8**)

### 3.2 TCR Transgenic Models of Passive EAE

The use of TCR transgenic mice can negate the requirement for immunization of donor mice and allows for simplified experimental variation in the conditions under which the T cells receive their initial activation. In addition, the resulting transferred population is a pure antigen-reactive cohort whereas, even after in vitro antigen-restimulation, populations from immunized WT mice will contain contaminating antigen-irrelevant cells.

There are various strains of TCR transgenic mice with CD4+ T cells specific for myelin-derived peptides (Table 1). Activated pathogenic T cells from myelin-reactive TCR transgenic mice are capable of inducing EAE upon transfer into MHC-syngeneic WT or RAG-deficient recipients [3, 4, 11]. In this section we describe the use of MBP(Ac1–9)-reactive cells from Tg4 mice [12], and their transfer into B10.PL or C57BL/6xB10.PL $F_1$ hosts. These methods should be applicable to other (but not necessarily all) myelin-reactive TCR transgenic strains, although note that the myelin peptide (Table 1) and (possibly) the concentration required during polarization will vary between the strains used.

The majority of protocols using TCR transgenic T cells to induce disease involve in vitro activation of naïve T cells (as described here), but cells from immunized TCR transgenic mice can also be used.

#### 3.2.1 Passive EAE Using TCR Transgenic Th1 Cells [3]

1. Remove spleens and peripheral LN from TCR transgenic mice and create a single cell suspension (Subheading 3.1.2, **steps 2–5**)
2. Culture cells at $4 \times 10^6$/ml in RPMI-10 % containing 10 μg/ml myelin peptide, 10 U/ml rIL-2, 25 ng/ml rIL-12, and 25 ng/ml rIL-18 in 6-well plates (4–6 ml per well) at 37 °C, 5 % $CO_2$ in a humidified atmosphere
3. After 48 h, split the cells and increase the concentration of IL-2 to 20 U/ml for the final 24 h
4. At the end of culture, process cells (Subheading 3.1.2, **steps 8–10**) and inject $3 \times 10^6$ blasts in a total volume of 200 μl PBS i.v. into WT hosts
5. In addition, inject 200 ng PTx in 500 μl PBS i.p. on the same day as cell transfer

#### 3.2.2 Passive EAE Using TCR Transgenic Th17 Cells (Adapted from Jager et al. [4])

1. Remove spleens and peripheral LN from TCR transgenic mice and create a single cell suspension (Subheading 3.1.2, **steps 2–5**)
2. Culture cells at $4 \times 10^6$/ml in RPMI-10 % containing 10 μg/ml myelin peptide, 30 ng/ml rIL-6, 3 ng/ml rTGF-β, 10 ng/ml rIL-1α, and 10 μg/ml anti-IFNγ in 6-well plates (4–6 ml per well) at 37 °C, 5 % $CO_2$ in a humidified atmosphere
3. After 48 h, split the cells with RPMI-10 % containing 10 ng/ml rIL-23, and transfer to vented T75 flasks
4. At day four/five assess visually and split if required with RPMI-10 %
5. Harvest the cells at day 6 and centrifuge at $350 \times g$ for 5 min

6. Resuspend cell pellets in wash buffer (10 ml per flask of cells) and purify live cells by separation over a Ficoll gradient (as per manufacturer's instructions)
7. Remove cells from the interface and wash in wash buffer
8. Culture cells at $1.5 \times 10^6$/ml in RPMI-10 % in 6-well plates (4–6 ml per well) coated with plate bound anti-CD3 and anti-CD28 (both at 2 μg/ml)
9. After 48 h process cells (Subheading 3.1.2, **steps 8–10**) and inject $5 \times 10^6$ blasts in a total volume of 200 μl PBS i.v. into WT hosts

#### 3.2.3 Passive EAE Using TCR Transgenic GM-CSF Producing Cells (Adapted from Codarri et al. [5])

1. Immunize myelin-reactive TCR transgenic mice with myelin peptide in CFA (Subheading 3.1.1)
2. Harvest and process cells (Subheading 3.1.2, **steps 1–5**)
3. Culture cells at $4 \times 10^6$/ml in RPMI-10 % containing myelin peptide, 10 μg/ml anti-IL-12, and 10 μg/ml anti-IFNγ
4. After 72 h process cells (Subheading 3.1.2, **steps 8–10**) and inject $5 \times 10^6$ lymphocytes in a total volume of 200 μl PBS i.v. into WT hosts

### 3.3 Clinical Evaluation of Disease

For all of the described methods of passive EAE induction, assess clinical signs of EAE from day 5 after cell transfer (Fig. 1).

Classical EAE [13]:

0—No disease

1—Flaccid tail

2—Impaired righting reflex and/or abnormal gait

3—Partial hind limb paralysis

4—Total hind limb paralysis

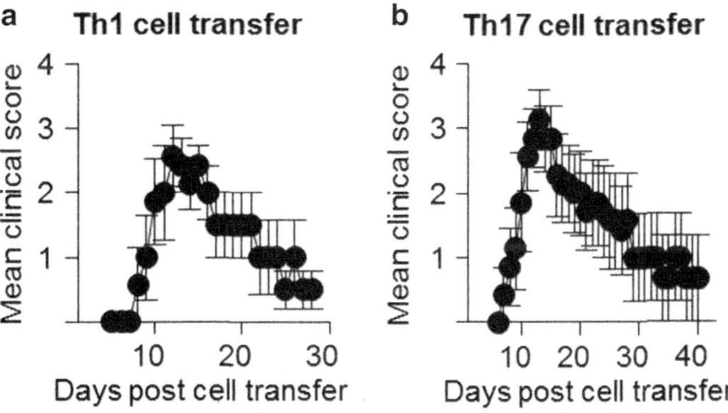


**Fig. 1** Clinical course of passive EAE (classical signs) induced by Th1- and Th17-polarized myelin-responsive T cells

5—Partial forelimb paralysis

6—Moribund or dead

Atypical disease (adapted from Stromnes et al. [14]):

0—No disease

1—Head tilted/slightly hunched appearance

2—Head tilt more pronounced/ataxia/scruffy coat

3—Body tilted and inability to walk in a straight line

4—Lying on side or involuntary and continuous rotation

5—Moribund or dead

The classical or atypical clinical manifestations of EAE appear to relate to the site of entry of pathogenic cells into the CNS. Atypical disease is more often seen in IL-23-conditioned or Th17 EAE models or those using IFN-γ-deficient T cells, where the cells preferentially enter the brain and cause inflammatory lesions in the brain stem and cerebellum [6, 14–16]. In contrast, classical EAE is associated predominantly with inflammatory cell entry into the spinal cord and is more often seen in passive EAE using IL-12 conditioned, or Th1 cells [17–19].

### 3.4 Phenotypic and Functional Analysis of Pathogenic T Cells

This section outlines the procedure for phenotypic analysis of cells at the end of polarizing culture and/or upon retrieval from mice. Table 2 states the expected phenotypic profiles for cells subjected to the Th1/IL-12 and Th17/IL-23 polarization culture, and Fig. 2 illustrates intracellular cytokine staining of polarized cells. Production of IFN-γ, IL-17, GM-CSF, and TNF-α can also be assessed by detection of these cytokines in the supernatant of cell cultures using Ready-SET-Go! ELISA sets (according to manufacturer's instructions).

**Table 2**
**Phenotypic characteristics of Th1/IL-12 conditioned and Th17/IL-23 conditioned T cells**

| | Phenotypic marker | Th1/IL-12 conditioned | Th17/IL-23 conditioned |
|---|---|---|---|
| Transcription factors | T-bet | ++ | – |
| | RORγt | – | ++ |
| Intracellular cytokines | IFN-γ | ++ | + |
| | IL-17 | + | ++ |
| | GM-CSF | + | + |
| | TNF-α | + | ++ |
| Chemokine receptors | CXCR3 | + | – |
| | CCR5 | + | – |
| | CCR6 | – | + |

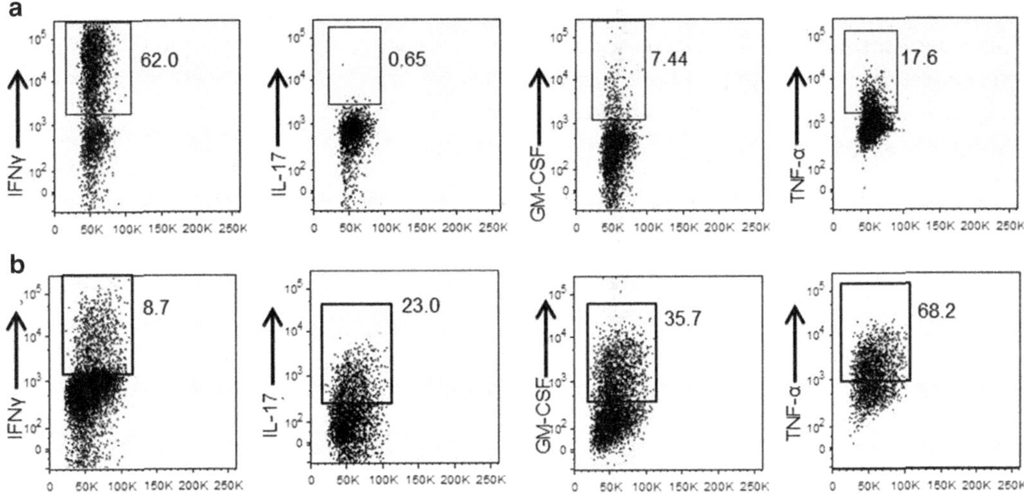


**Fig. 2** Intracellular cytokine staining for Th1-polarized (**a**) and Th17-polarized (**b**) myelin-responsive T cells on the day of cell transfer

1. For samples where intracellular cytokine staining is not required, proceed directly to **step 4**.
2. For cytokine analysis of donor cells retrieved from mice, culture cells in RPMI-10 % overnight with the appropriate myelin-derived peptide and add 1 μl/ml brefeldin A for the last 4 h of culture.
3. For cytokine analysis of cells at the end of polarization, add 50 ng/ml PMA, 50 ng/ml ionomycin and 1 μl/ml brefeldin A to an aliquot of cells for the last 4 h of culture.
4. Wash the cells twice in PBS and stain cells with fixable viability dye in PBS according to manufacturer's instructions.
5. Wash the cells twice in FACS buffer and surface-stain with the relevant antibody (anti-CD4, antibodies to congenic marker, if retrieved donor cells express an appropriate distinguishing marker) in FACS buffer for 20 min (*see* **Note 9**).
6. Wash cells in FACS buffer and process for intracellular staining using proprietary fix/perm buffers according to the manufacturer's instructions (e-Bioscience for transcription factor staining or BD Biosciences for cytokine staining).
7. Stain for intracellular antigens in the indicated permeabilization buffers and with the relevant antibodies (Subheading 2).
8. Wash and resuspend cells in FACS buffer and keep at 4 °C in the dark until acquired.

### *3.5 Isolation of Mononuclear Cells from the CNS (Adapted from McGeachy et al. [20])*

Pathogenic T cells can be identified in the CNS from the onset of clinical disease until the later stages of the resolution phase. The phenotypic characteristics of these cells can be determined by flow cytometry (Subheading 3.4).

1. Cull mice by $CO_2$ asphyxiation.
2. Perfuse the mice transcardially via the left ventricle with 10 ml cold PBS
3. Dissect out the vertebral column and remove the spinal cord by intrathecal hydrostatic pressure using 1 ml cold PBS; place in wash buffer.
4. Remove brain by dissection and place in wash buffer.
5. Cut the brain and spinal cord into small pieces and manually disaggregate using a 1 ml syringe.
6. Digest the brain and spinal cord in 400 μl digestion buffer for 40 min at 37 °C.
7. Isolate mononuclear cells using a 30:70 % discontinuous Percoll gradient and centrifugation at 530×*g* for 20 min; cells can be obtained from the interface.
8. Resuspend cells at $4 \times 10^6$/ml in RPMI-10 % and process cells for phenotypic analysis (Subheading 3.4).

## 4 Notes

1. The concentration of *M. tuberculosis* in the adjuvant used varies between protocols. The concentration of *M. tuberculosis* in purchased CFA is 1 mg/ml (Sigma). If a higher concentration of *M. tuberculosis* is required this can be achieved through the addition of *M. tuberculosis* H37Ra (nonviable, desiccated) (VWR International, UK) to an appropriate volume of incomplete Freund's adjuvant (IFA).
2. MOG (35–55) has a C-terminal COOH group. MBP Ac1–9 requires a C-terminal amide group to maintain antigenicity.
3. Donor mice can be immunized with spinal cord homogenate, purified or recombinant myelin proteins or synthetic peptides containing known T cell epitopes (Table 1). Antigen is mixed with adjuvant to provide prolonged stimulation; we find that CFA is most effective, but some groups report the use of IFA [10].
4. Some groups report the addition of anti-IL-4 at 10 μg/ml and recombinant IFNγ at 2 ng/ml [10].
5. Some protocols sort CD4+ cells at the end of culture to ensure pure transfer or use CD4 purity staining to normalize the number of cells transferred [6, 7, 10]. We have found that sorting is not necessary as purity tends to be high (above 80 %).

6. The number of cells to transfer for pathogenicity will need to be optimized accordingly for different cells and host strains.
7. Cell culture volume will need to be optimized. However, we do not recommend culturing in larger flasks as viability is reduced.
8. IL-23 conditioned cells can be administered i.v. or i.p. Robust EAE can be successfully established using either route of injection.
9. For identification of transferred donor cells using congenic markers, surface-stain for CD45.1/2 or CD90.1/2 as appropriate.

## References


1. Ben-Nun A, Wekerle H, Cohen IR (1981) The rapid isolation of clonable antigen-specific T lymphocyte lines capable of mediating autoimmune encephalomyelitis. Eur J Immunol 11(3):195–199
2. Zamvil S et al (1985) T-cell clones specific for myelin basic protein induce chronic relapsing paralysis and demyelination. Nature 317(6035): 355–358
3. O'Connor RA et al (2008) Cutting edge: Th1 cells facilitate the entry of Th17 cells to the central nervous system during experimental autoimmune encephalomyelitis. J Immunol 181(6):3750–3754
4. Jager A et al (2009) Th1, Th17, and Th9 effector cells induce experimental autoimmune encephalomyelitis with different pathological phenotypes. J Immunol 183(11):7169–7177
5. Codarri L et al (2011) RORgammat drives production of the cytokine GM-CSF in helper T cells, which is essential for the effector phase of autoimmune neuroinflammation. Nat Immunol 12(6):560–567
6. Kroenke MA, Chensue SW, Segal BM (2010) EAE mediated by a non-IFN-gamma/non-IL-17 pathway. Eur J Immunol 40(8):2340–2348
7. Kroenke MA, Segal BM (2011) IL-23 modulated myelin-specific T cells induce EAE via an IFNgamma driven, IL-17 independent pathway. Brain Behav Immun 25(5):932–937
8. O'Connor RA, Malpass KH, Anderton SM (2007) The inflamed central nervous system drives the activation and rapid proliferation of Foxp3+ regulatory T cells. J Immunol 179(2): 958–966
9. Ito A et al (2003) Transfer of severe experimental autoimmune encephalomyelitis by IL-12- and IL-18-potentiated T cells is estrogen sensitive. J Immunol 170(9):4802–4809
10. Kroenke MA et al (2008) IL-12- and IL-23-modulated T cells induce distinct types of EAE based on histology, CNS chemokine profile, and response to cytokine inhibition. J Exp Med 205(7):1535–1541
11. Ghoreschi K et al (2010) Generation of pathogenic T(H)17 cells in the absence of TGF-beta signalling. Nature 467(7318):967–971
12. Liu GY et al (1995) Low avidity recognition of self-antigen by T cells permits escape from central tolerance. Immunity 3(4):407–415
13. Ryan KR, McCue D, Anderton SM (2005) Fas-mediated death and sensory adaptation limit the pathogenic potential of autoreactive T cells after strong antigenic stimulation. J Leukoc Biol 78(1):43–50
14. Stromnes IM et al (2008) Differential regulation of central nervous system autoimmunity by T(H)1 and T(H)17 cells. Nat Med 14(3): 337–342
15. Wensky AK et al (2005) IFN-gamma determines distinct clinical outcomes in autoimmune encephalomyelitis. J Immunol 174(3): 1416–1423
16. Rothhammer V et al (2011) Th17 lymphocytes traffic to the central nervous system independently of alpha4 integrin expression during EAE. J Exp Med 208(12):2465–2476
17. Muller DM, Pender MP, Greer JM (2000) A neuropathological analysis of experimental autoimmune encephalomyelitis with predominant brain stem and cerebellar involvement and differences between active and passive induction. Acta Neuropathol 100(2): 174–182
18. Lees JR et al (2008) Regional CNS responses to IFN-gamma determine lesion localization patterns during EAE pathogenesis. J Exp Med 205(11):2633–2642

19. Domingues HS et al (2010) Functional and pathogenic differences of Th1 and Th17 cells in experimental autoimmune encephalomyelitis. PLoS One 5(11):e15531
20. McGeachy MJ, Stephens LA, Anderton SM (2005) Natural recovery and protection from autoimmune encephalomyelitis: contribution of CD4+CD25+ regulatory cells within the central nervous system. J Immunol 175(5): 3025–3032
21. Lafaille JJ et al (1994) High incidence of spontaneous autoimmune encephalomyelitis in immunodeficient anti-myelin basic protein T cell receptor transgenic mice. Cell 78(3): 399–408
22. Zamvil SS et al (1985) Encephalitogenic T cell clones specific for myelin basic protein. An unusual bias in antigen recognition. J Exp Med 162(6):2107–2124
23. Goverman J et al (1993) Transgenic mice that express a myelin basic protein-specific T cell receptor develop spontaneous autoimmunity. Cell 72(4):551–560
24. Hardardottir F, Baron JL, Janeway CA Jr (1995) T cells with two functional antigen-specific receptors. Proc Natl Acad Sci U S A 92(2):354–358
25. Sakai K et al (1988) Characterization of a major encephalitogenic T cell epitope in SJL/J mice with synthetic oligopeptides of myelin basic protein. J Neuroimmunol 19(1–2):21–32
26. Tuohy V et al (1989) Identification of an encephalitogenic determinant of myelin proteolipid protein for SJL mice. J Immunol 142(5):1523–1527
27. Waldner H et al (2000) Fulminant spontaneous autoimmunity of the central nervous system in mice transgenic for the myelin proteolipid protein-specific T cell receptor. Proc Natl Acad Sci U S A 97(7):3412–3417
28. Greer JM et al (1992) Identification and characterization of a second encephalitogenic determinant of myelin proteolipid protein (residues 178-191) for SJL mice. J Immunol 149(3): 783–788
29. Amor S et al (1993) Identification of a major encephalitogenic epitope of proteolipid protein (residues 56-70) for the induction of experimental allergic encephalomyelitis in Biozzi AB/H and nonobese diabetic mice. J Immunol 150(12):5666–5672
30. Amor S et al (1994) Identification of epitopes of myelin oligodendrocyte glycoprotein for the induction of experimental allergic encephalomyelitis in SJL and Biozzi AB/H mice. J Immunol 153(10):4349–4356
31. Mendel I, de Rosbo NK, Ben-Nun A (1995) A myelin oligodendrocyte glycoprotein peptide induces typical chronic experimental autoimmune encephalomyelitis in H-2b mice: fine specificity and T cell receptor Vβ expression of encephalitogenic T cells. Eur J Immunol 25(7): 1951–1959
32. Bettelli E et al (2003) Myelin oligodendrocyte glycoprotein-specific T cell receptor transgenic mice develop spontaneous autoimmune optic neuritis. J Exp Med 197(9):1073–1081
33. de Rosbo NK, Mendel I, Ben-Nun A (1995) Chronic relapsing experimental autoimmune encephalomyelitis with a delayed onset and an atypical clinical course, induced in PL/J mice by myelin oligodendrocyte glycoprotein (MOG)-derived peptide: preliminary analysis of MOG T cell epitopes. Eur J Immunol 25(4):985–993

# Chapter 18

# Experimental Mouse Models of T Cell-Dependent Inflammatory Bowel Disease

**George X. Song-Zhao and Kevin J. Maloy**

## Abstract

Inflammatory bowel diseases (IBD) represent idiopathic chronic inflammatory disorders of the intestinal tract that are associated with aberrant immune responses against intestinal bacteria. Here, we describe two T cell-dependent models of experimental murine IBD. In the "T cell transfer" model, lymphopenic (*scid* or *Rag*$^{-/-}$) mice develop colitis upon adoptive transfer of naïve CD4$^{+}$ T cells. This model has also been extensively employed to identify mechanisms through which CD4$^{+}$CD25$^{+}$ regulatory T cells suppress intestinal inflammation in vivo. We also describe a model of T cell-dependent IBD in immunocompetent mice, induced by infection with the intestinal bacterium *Helicobacter hepaticus* and concomitant treatment with a blocking αIL-10R mAb, which leads to the development of chronic inflammation of the caecum and colon (typhlocolitis). Both models reproduce many facets of human IBD pathology, including epithelial hyperplasia, goblet cell depletion, and leukocyte infiltration. These models provide reliable and tractable systems for the analyses of the induction and regulation of chronic inflammation in the gut.

**Key words** Mucosal immunology, Inflammatory bowel disease, Colitis, T cells, *Helicobacter hepaticus*

## 1 Introduction

Crohn's disease (CD) and ulcerative colitis (UC) represent the two major clinical forms of inflammatory bowel disease (IBD), debilitating chronic inflammatory disorders of the intestinal tract [1]. Although disease etiology is incompletely understood, pathology is mediated by dysregulated host immune responses to the intestinal microbiota [2]. A variety of spontaneous and induced mouse models of IBD have been developed, which have contributed to an improved understanding of the pathogenesis of intestinal inflammation [1–5]. A number of these models have identified T cell function as central to intestinal homeostasis, with distinct subsets of CD4$^{+}$ T cells associated with either induction or regulation of

Ari Waisman and Burkhard Becher (eds.), *T-Helper Cells: Methods and Protocols*, Methods in Molecular Biology, vol. 1193, DOI 10.1007/978-1-4939-1212-4_18, © Springer Science+Business Media New York 2014

intestinal inflammation [1, 2, 6]. In this chapter, we describe two well-characterized T cell-dependent mouse IBD models that have been employed to further characterize the role of T cells in intestinal pathology.

The 'T cell transfer' colitis model was established by Powrie et al. [7], who found that upon adoptive transfer of naïve $CD4^{+}CD45RB^{high}$ T cells into immunodeficient hosts, such as *Rag*$^{-/-}$ or severe combined immunodeficiency (*scid*) mice, the T cells dramatically expanded and differentiated in the intestine in response to components of the microbiota [8, 9]. This resulted in inflammation of the entire large intestine with characteristic histological features of IBD, such as depletion of goblet cells, leukocyte infiltration, ulcerations, and crypt abscesses [8–11]. This model has been instrumental in defining cellular and molecular pathways that mediate chronic intestinal inflammation, such as the recent demonstration that IL-23 plays a key role in driving pathogenic Th1 and Th17 responses in the gut [12, 13]. In addition to identifying pathogenic circuits, the T cell transfer IBD model was crucial for demonstrating the immunosuppressive function of $CD4^{+}CD25^{+}$ regulatory T cells (Treg), which can both prevent and cure chronic intestinal inflammation [6, 14].

One caveat of the T cell transfer model is that it involves lymphopenic immunodeficient hosts, which are prone to infection and which have some abnormalities in lymphoid architecture. In addition, the precise components of the intestinal microflora that drive activation and expansion of pathogenic T cell responses are not well characterized. However, when combined with infection with the murine intestinal bacteria *Helicobacter hepaticus*, the T cell transfer model demonstrated the ability of a single bacterial species to exacerbate colitis [15]. Indeed, *H. hepaticus* has been found to induce chronic intestinal inflammation in several genetically susceptible hosts, particularly those with perturbations in immune regulatory factors [16]. In contrast, in wild-type mice persistent *H. hepaticus* infection does not result in colitis, due to the induction of specific Treg cells that secrete IL-10 [17]. However, this dominant Treg response can be overcome through blockade of IL-10R using monoclonal antibodies, revealing the presence of potent *H. hepaticus*-specific Th1 and Th17 responses that induce chronic typhlocolitis (inflammation in both the caecum and colon) [18]. Therefore, the *H. hepaticus*-induced T cell-mediated IBD allows for the investigation of chronic intestinal inflammation in the context of a defined bacterial infection. Another advantage of this model is the ability to induce IBD in non-genetically manipulated wild-type mice under physiological conditions where no immune cell populations are missing.

## 2 Materials

### 2.1 Mice

The T cell transfer IBD model requires wild-type $CD4^+$ T cell donor mice and syngeneic immunodeficient recipient mice. This model has been successfully carried out on various inbred mouse strains with distinct genetic backgrounds (*see* **Note 1**).

The *Helicobacter hepaticus* plus anti-IL-10R IBD model is performed in wild-type C57BL/6 mice.

Since changes in microbiota or the presence of intestinal pathogens have been found to affect disease outcome [15, 19, 20], it is important that all mice are housed under specific pathogen free (SPF) conditions (*see* **Notes 2** and **3**).

### 2.2 Reagents for T Cell Transfer Colitis

1. BSA buffer: PBS + 0.1 % BSA.
2. 2 mL disposable syringes.
3. Sterile cell strainers (100 μm; BD Biosciences, Cat. No. 352360).
4. 50 mL conical tubes.
5. ACK lysis buffer: 0.15 M $NH_4Cl$, 10 mM $KHCO_3$, 0.1 mM $Na_2EDTA$, adjust pH to 7.2 with 1 M HCl.
6. CD4 enrichment antibody cocktail (prepare each antibody for a final concentration of 10 μg/mL in BSA buffer): αB220 (clone RA3-6B2), αCD11b (αMac-1, clone M1/70), αCD8 (clone YTS169), αMHCII (clone TIB120) (*see* **Note 4**).
7. Dynabeads® Sheep Anti-Rat IgG (Life Technologies, Cat. No. 11035), Dynabeads® MPC®-1 (Magnetic Particle Processor) (Life Technologies, Cat. No. 12001D).
8. 14 mL polystyrene round-bottom tubes.
9. FACS staining reagents: Viability Dye eFluor® 780 (eBioscience Cat. No. 65-0865), CD4-APC (clone RM4-5; eBioscience, Cat. No. 17-0042-82) CD45RB-FITC (clone C363.16A; BD Biosciences, Cat. No. 553100), CD25-PE (clone 7D4; BD Biosciences, Cat. No. 558642).
10. 5 mL polypropylene FACS tubes with lid.
11. FCS buffer: PBS + 10 % FCS + 2 mM EDTA.
12. Electronic balance.
13. Dissection scissors, curved forceps, scalpel.
14. Formal saline: PBS + 3.6 % (w/v) formaldehyde.

### 2.3 Reagents for *H. hepaticus*-Induced Colitis

1. QIAamp DNA Stool Mini Kit (Qiagen, Cat. No. 51504).
2. Primers for *H. hepaticus*-specific (p25) gene [21]. Forward primer: ATG GGT AAG AAA ATA GCA AAA AGA TTG CAA; reverse primer: CTA TTT CAT ATC CAT AAG CTC

TTG AGA ATC; annealing temperature: 55 °C; amplicon length: 705 bp.

3. Primers for pan-*Helicobacter* genus-specific (16S rRNA) [22]. Forward primer: GCT ATG ACG GGT ATC C; reverse primer: GAT TTT ACC CCT ACA CCA; annealing temperature: 58 °C; amplicon length: 422 bp.
4. Blood agar plates: dissolve 40 g/L of Blood Agar Base No 2 (Oxoid, Cat. No. CM0271) in water and autoclave. After autoclaving, cool agar to 50 °C and add 4 μL/mL Campylobacter Selective Supplement (TVP; Oxoid, Cat. No. SR0069E) and 75 μL/mL Laked Horse Blood (Oxoid, Cat. No. SR0048C). Pour prepared agar into disposable petri dishes (*see* **Note 5**).
5. Tryptic Soy Broth (TSB) media: dissolve 30 g/L of TSB powder (Oxoid, Cat. No. CM0129) in water and autoclave. Allow to cool and add 10 % FCS and 4 μL/mL Campylobacter Selective Supplement before use.
6. 250 mL sterile ventilated disposable flasks (Thermo, Cat. No. 4116-0250).
7. Anaerobic jar (Oxoid, Cat. No. HP0011A).
8. Vacuum pump.
9. Anaerobic gas mixture: 80 % $N_2$, 10 % $CO_2$, 10 % $H_2$ (BOC, Cat. No. 290564-L).
10. Viability stain: LIVE/DEAD® BacLight™ Bacterial Viability Kit (Life Technologies, Cat. No. L7012). Working solution is then prepared by diluting the stock solution at 1/1,000 with water, aliquot, and store at 4 °C in microtubes covered in aluminum foil.
11. Feeding needles (Cadence Science, 22G, Cat. No. 7920) and 1 mL disposable syringes for oral gavage.
12. BSA buffer: PBS + 0.1 % BSA.
13. Microcentrifuge tubes.
14. Electronic balance.
15. Dissection scissors, curved forceps, scalpel.
16. Chromatography paper (Whatman, Cat. No. 3030-861).
17. Formol saline: PBS + 3.6 % (w/v) formaldehyde.
18. *H. hepaticus* genomic DNA: isolated using the DNeasy Blood & Tissue Kit (Qiagen, Cat. No. 69504).
19. Primers for *H. hepaticus* ctdB gene were designed according to Ge et al. [23]. Forward primer: CCG CAA ATT GCA GCA ATA CTT; reverse primer: TCG TCC AAA ATG CAC AGG TG; probe: AAT ATA CGC GCA CAC CTC TCA TCT GAC CAT.

## 3 Methods

### 3.1 T Cell Transfer Colitis

All steps performed below (*see* Fig. 1) should be kept sterile using sterile equipment and reagents

#### 3.1.1 Spleen Cell Isolation

1. Isolate spleens from mice and place into BSA buffer and store on ice. Each spleen should yield approximately $1 \times 10^6$ naïve $CD4^+CD25^-CD45RB^{high}$ T cells and $2 \times 10^5$ $CD4^+CD25^+CD45RB^-$ Treg cells.
2. Obtain single cells by grinding spleens through a cell strainer into a 50 mL conical tube using the plunger of a disposable syringe. Up to 5 spleens can be pooled in each 50 mL tube.
3. Rinse the strainer with 10 mL of BSA buffer and pipette repeatedly to break up any cell aggregates in the 50 mL conical tube.

#### 3.1.2 Red Blood Cell Lysis

1. Centrifuge at $400 \times g$ for 5 min to pellet cells. Aspirate supernatant and thoroughly resuspend pellet in ACK lysis buffer (1 mL per spleen) and incubate for 3 min at room temperature (*see* **Note 6**).

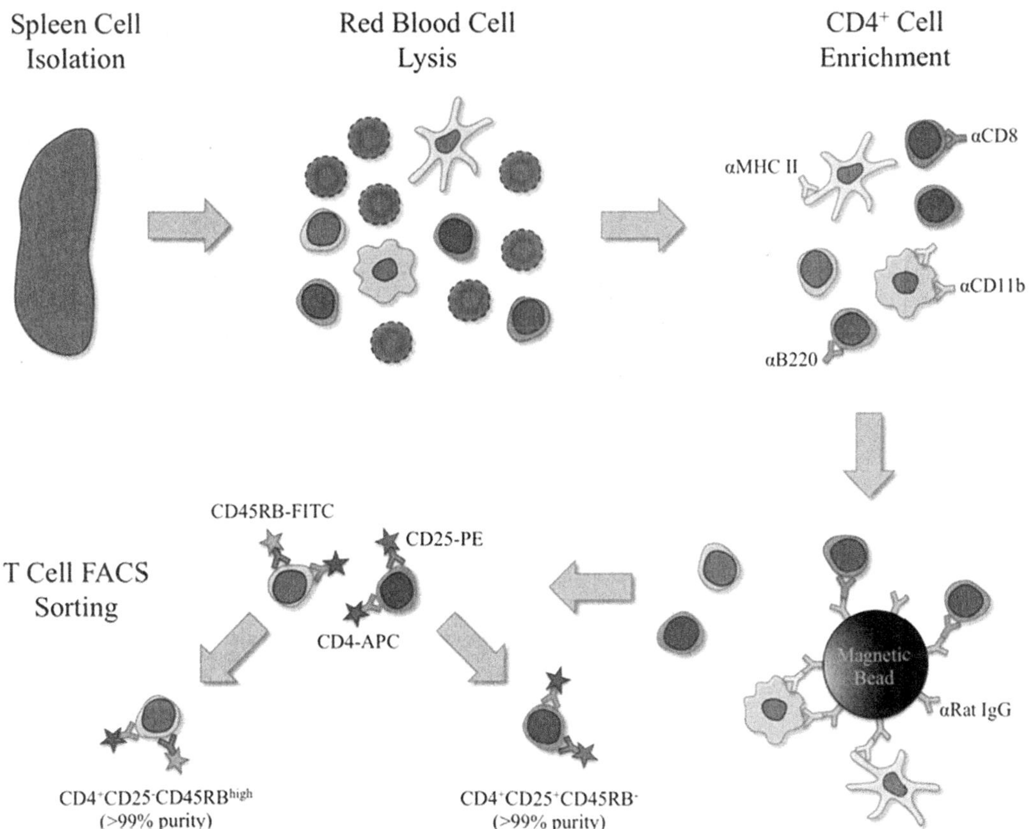


**Fig. 1** Summary of $CD4^+$ T-cell isolation

2. Add 10 mL of BSA buffer per spleen and filter through a cell strainer into a fresh 50 mL conical tube.
3. Remove a 100 μL aliquot and count viable cells with a hemocytometer. Pellet the remaining cells in the 50 mL tube by centrifugation at 400 × *g* for 5 min and aspirate supernatant.

#### 3.1.3 CD4+ Cell Enrichment

1. Resuspend isolated cell pellet in CD4 enrichment antibody cocktail (use 50 μL per $10^7$ cells) and incubate at 4 °C for 20 min. Wash by adding 20 mL BSA buffer then pellet cells by centrifugation at 400 × *g* for 5 min and aspirate supernatant. Resuspend cells at $1 \times 10^8$ per mL in BSA buffer.
2. Thoroughly resuspend Dynabeads® Sheep Anti-Rat IgG beads in the stock bottle and remove the amount required to yield a 1:1 (beads–cells) ratio and add to a 14 mL polystyrene round-bottom tube.
3. Wash beads by adding 5 mL BSA buffer and mixing, then leave in the Magnetic Particle Processor for 30 s. Discard wash by aspirating using a 5 mL pipette to avoid touching the beads. Repeat washing process with 5 mL fresh BSA buffer.
4. Resuspend beads at $1 \times 10^8$ per mL in BSA buffer and add to cells (also resuspended at $1 \times 10^8$ per mL). Incubate on a rotary mixer at 4 °C for 20 min.
5. To separate cells, place tube on Magnetic Particle Processor for 30 s and recover the supernatant, which contains the CD4-enriched cells, into a fresh 15 mL centrifuge tube. Repeat magnetic selection to remove any remaining beads.
6. Add 5 volumes of BSA buffer, pellet cells in a centrifuge at 400 × *g* for 5 min and count cells using a hemocytometer.

#### 3.1.4 T Cell FACS Sorting

1. Resuspend cells at $1 \times 10^8$ cells/mL in BSA buffer. Remove aliquots of $5 \times 10^5$ cells as staining controls for cell sorting (*see* **Note 7**). Stain CD4-enriched cells with Viability Dye eFluor® 780 (1:1,000), 1 μg/mL CD4-APC, 2.5 μg/mL CD45RB-FITC, and 1 μg/mL CD25-PE. Mix well and incubate at 4 °C for 20 min in the dark.
2. Wash cells with 10 mL BSA buffer and pellet cells by centrifugation at 400 × *g* for 5 min. Resuspend cell pellet in another 10 mL BSA buffer and filter through a cell strainer to remove cell aggregates to prevent blocking of the cell sorter. Finally pellet cells by centrifugation at 400 × *g* for 5 min and resuspend cells at 2–5 × $10^7$ cells/mL in FCS buffer for sorting.
3. Using a FACS machine (*see* **Note 7**) separate the $CD4^+CD25^-CD45RB^{high}$ naïve T cells and $CD4^+CD25^+CD45RB^-$ Treg cells (if required) using appropriate sorting gates (*see* Fig. 2). Cells should be collected into 5 mL polypropylene FACS tubes with lid containing 100 μL of heat-inactivated FCS and stored on ice.

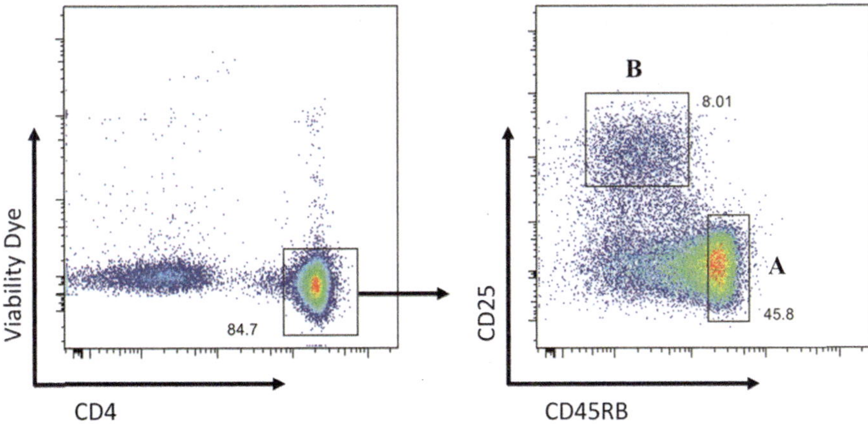


**Fig. 2** Gating strategy for FACS sorting of CD4⁺ T cells. The *left hand panel* shows a typical gate to select viable CD4⁺ T cells, which are then separated into different subpopulations using the gates shown on the *right hand panel*; $CD4^+CD25^-CD45RB^{high}$ naïve T cells (A) and $CD4^+CD25^+CD45RB^-$ Treg cells (B, approximately 90 % should be $Foxp3^+$)

4. Centrifuge sorted fractions at $400 \times g$ for 5 min to pellet the cells and determine cell numbers using a hemocytometer.
5. Verify the purity of sorted populations FACS by reanalyzing about $1 \times 10^5$ cells from each fraction. Purity should be >99 %.

#### 3.1.5 Colitis Induction

1. Pellet the purified CD4+ T cell populations by centrifuging at $400 \times g$ for 5 min. Resuspend $CD4^+CD45RB^{high}$ naïve T cells at $4 \times 10^6$/mL and the $CD4^+CD25^+CD45RB^-$ Treg cells at $1 \times 10^6$/mL.
2. To induce T cell transfer IBD, inject $4 \times 10^5$ $CD4^+CD45RB^{high}$ naïve T cells (100 μL) intraperitoneally into a syngeneic *Rag*$^{-/-}$ recipient mouse.
   To protect from disease, inject $4 \times 10^5$ $CD4^+CD25^-CD45RB^{high}$ naïve T cells (100 μL) together with $1 \times 10^5$ $CD4^+CD25^+CD45RB^-$ Treg cells (100 μL) intraperitoneally into a syngeneic *Rag*$^{-/-}$ recipient mouse.
3. Identify each mouse by ear punching in order to keep track of different treatment groups.

#### 3.1.6 Disease Monitoring and Assessment

1. Weigh and monitor animals weekly for weight loss, hunching, loose stools/diarrhea, and/or scruffy coat. Once symptoms are present, mice should be observed on a daily basis (*see* **Note 8**).
2. Sacrifice mice once they exhibit chronic diarrhea or when they drop to 80–90 % of their initial body weight. The time until the onset of disease is facility-dependent, severe colitis normally occurs at around 6–8 weeks, but may occur at any time point between 4 and 12 weeks.

3. Open abdomen, dissect out the entire colon, place lengthwise on a piece of paper towel moistened with PBS, and trim away any attached mesentery and fat. Use a scalpel to cut 5–7 mm pieces of proximal, mid, and distal colon (*see* **Note 9**) and gently remove luminal contents using the back of curved forceps.
4. Fix tissue pieces in 10 mL of formal saline for at least 24 h. Samples should be sent to a histology lab for histological processing and staining. Samples should be embedded in paraffin and 4–5 μm cross sections cut and mounted onto glass slides for staining with hematoxylin and eosin (H and E), with 2–3 sections prepared per sample.
5. Stained histological sample slides should be assessed in a blinded fashion according to the semi-quantitative scoring scheme described in Table 1 [24]. For each category (epithelium, inflammation in lamina propria, area affected, and markers of severe inflammation) a score should be given between 0 and 3, resulting in a total score for each colon section sample of 0–12.
6. For each mouse, scores from proximal, mid, and distal colon sections should be averaged to give a mean overall colitis score. Differences between treatment groups should be analyzed using a nonparametric statistical test (e.g. Mann Whitney).

### 3.2 Helicobacter hepaticus-Induced T Cell-Dependent IBD

#### 3.2.1 H. hepaticus Screening

1. Collect fecal pellets from mice into PBS and extract DNA using the QIAamp DNA Stool Mini Kit.
2. Perform PCR using primers designed to amplify either *H. hepaticus*-specific (p25) or pan-*Helicobacter* genus-specific (16S rRNA) genes.
3. Determine PCR products on a 1.5 % agarose gel.

#### 3.2.2 H. hepaticus Culturing

1. *H. hepaticus* NCI-Frederick isolate 1A (ATCC strain 51449) should be grown either on blood agar plates or in TSB media at 37 °C under microaerophilic conditions (*see* **Note 10**).
2. 1 mL of TSB media should be prepared for every 5 plates of *H. hepaticus* to be harvested (at least 1 mL of media needed in order to submerge the tip of the cotton swab).
3. To harvest, dip the sterile cotton swab into TSB and rub along the surface of the plate, and then spin the swab in TSB to release collected bacteria
4. To confirm the viability of the harvested bacteria, add about 5–10 μL of harvested bacteria to 50 μL of Viability stain (*see* **Note 11**).

#### 3.2.3 Disease Induction

1. Estimate concentration of bacterial culture with the following equation: 1 $OD_{600} = 1 \times 10^8$ CFU/mL
2. Centrifuge to pellet bacteria and resuspend to $5 \times 10^8$ CFU/mL in sterile PBS and infect by oral gavage of 0.2 mL

**Table 1**
**Summary of histological scoring colitis**

| | | | | | | |
|---|---|---|---|---|---|---|
| A | Epithelium | Hyperplasia | and/or | Goblet cell depletion | | |
| | 0 | None | | None | | |
| | 1 | Mild (1.5×) | | Mild (25 %) | | |
| | 2 | Moderate (2–3×) | | Marked (25–50 %) | | |
| | 3 | Severe (>3×) | | Substantial (>50 %) | | |
| B | Inflammation in lamina propria | | | | | |
| | 0 | None—few leucocytes | | | | |
| | 1 | Mild—some increase in leukocytes at tips of crypts OR many lymphoid follicles | | | | |
| | 2 | Moderate—marked infiltrate (notable broadening of crypt) | | | | |
| | 3 | Severe—dense infiltrate throughout | | | | |
| C | Area affected (% of section) | | | | | |
| | 0 | None | | | | |
| | 1 | Up to 25 % | | | | |
| | 2 | 25–50 % | | | | |
| | 3 | >50 % | | | | |
| D | Markers of severe inflammation | Submucosal inflammation | | Crypt abscesses | Crypt branching | Ulceration OR extensive fibrosis |
| | 0 | None | | None | None | None |
| | 1 | Mild | OR | Few (<5) | None | None |
| | 2 | Mild | AND | Few (<5) | None | None |
| | 2 | Extensive | OR | Many (>5) OR | Yes | None |
| | 3 | Extensive | AND | Many (>5) OR | Yes | None |
| | 3 | – | | – | – | Yes |

(1 × 10⁸ CFU/mouse) using a feeding needle on day 0, 1, and 2 to ensure successful infection.

3. Inject 1 mg αIL-10R mAb (clone: 1B1.2) i.p. on the first day of infection. The injection is repeated again on day 7, 14, and 21.

*3.2.4 Disease Monitoring and Assessment*

1. Weigh and observe animals weekly for weight loss, hunching, loose stools/diarrhea, and/or scruffy coat. Once symptoms are present, mice should be observed on a daily basis.
2. Sacrifice mice on day 28 post-infection.

3. Isolate the caecum, place into a microcentrifuge tube containing 1 mL of BSA buffer and shake vigorously to release caecal contents. Freeze caecal contents for determination of *H. hepaticus* colonization levels. Retrieve caecum out of the microcentrifuge tube and place (luminal side up) on a piece of chromatography paper (for support). Then fix caecum in formal saline and process sample according to **step 5**.
4. Isolate colon and trim away any attached mesentery and fat. Cut 5–7 mm pieces of proximal, mid, and distal colon and gently remove luminal contents using the back of curved forceps.
5. Fix caecum and colon tissue pieces in 10 mL of formal saline for 24 h. Following histological processing and staining, embed samples in paraffin and cut 4–5 μm cross sections for staining with hematoxylin and eosin (H and E).
6. Stained histological sample slides should be assessed in a blinded fashion according to the characteristics described in Table 1. For each category (epithelium, inflammation in lamina propria, area affected, and markers of severe inflammation) a score should be given between 0 and 3. Factors considered in each category are listed in Table 1.
7. Scores from affected colon section(s) should be averaged and any significant differences between treatment groups analyzed using a nonparametric statistical test (Mann–Whitney). Caecal scores should be tallied separately and also analyzed using the Mann–Whitney test.

#### 3.2.5 *H. hepaticus* Quantification

1. Isolate DNA from caecal content upon sacrifice of animals using the QIAamp DNA Stool Mini Kit.
2. Normalize amount of caecal DNA and perform quantitative PCR using primers and probes for *H. hepaticus* ctdB gene according to Ge et al. [23], using serial dilutions of *H. hepaticus* genomic DNA to generate a standard curve.

## 4 Notes

1. Although the kinetics and incidence may vary, the T cell transfer IBD model works well in most inbred immunodeficient strains, including C57BL/6.*Rag*$^{-/-}$ [25], BALB/c.*Rag*$^{-/-}$ [26], and C.B-17 SCID mice [7, 27]. In contrast, transfer of naïve CD4$^{+}$ T cells from 129SvEv into 129SvEv.*Rag*$^{-/-}$ mice only results in mild intestinal inflammation [28].
2. It is very important that mice are maintained under SPF conditions, as pathogens present in either recipient or donor mice can lead to confounding effects. This should be suspected if the immune deficient recipient strains develop rapid wasting

disease (within 2 weeks) after T cell transfer, which can be triggered by the presence of *Pneumocystis carinii* or viral infection. Until relatively recently, intestinal *Helicobacter* spp. were endemic in many animal facilities and since these can induce or impact disease severity in these IBD models, it is important that both donor and recipient strains are free from *Helicobacter* spp. To minimize the infection risk, it is advised that mice be housed in individually ventilated filter cages and regular pathogen screening of mouse colonies is performed.

3. The intestinal microbiota is probably the key determinant of the characteristics of T cell transfer IBD within a given animal facility and alterations in microbiota may affect the penetrance, severity and kinetics of disease. Therefore, antibiotics, or other agents that may affect the microbiota (such as chlorine tablets used to sterilize water), should be avoided where possible, or empirically titrated to ensure that disease induction is not affected.
4. Instead of the described CD4 enrichment antibody cocktail, a commercial isolation kit can also be used: Dynabeads® Untouched™ Mouse CD4 Cells (Life Technologies, Cat. No. 11415D)
5. Campylobacter Selective Supplement contains: 5 μg/mL trimethoprim, 10 μg/mL vancomycin, 25 IU/mL polymyxin B. Ensure that both the antibiotics and blood are at room temperature before addition to agar in order to prevent clumping. To test temperature of the agar, put a few drops of blood into the molten agar. If the agar is too hot then blood will turn black. At the right temperature the blood–agar mixture should remain transparent.
6. Do not incubate cells with ACK lysis buffer for longer than 3 min as prolonged incubation results in cell lysis. Store the ACK lysis buffer at room temperature, so that it does not need to be warmed up beforehand.
7. FACS sorting requires technical expertise and is normally performed by a highly trained operator. It is very important to discuss your aims and sorting strategy with the operator before you begin the experiment. They should be able to advise on staining controls to determine the correct compensations when setting up the FACS sorter—this may be either single stained control cell samples or standardized fluorescent beads. The operator should also be able to assist with defining optimal sorting gates for cell separation and with re-analyses of the sorted cell fractions. If possible, FACS sorting should be conducted under sterile conditions, using sterile running buffer and collection tubes.
8. Symptoms of colitis and wasting disease are usually evident by about 4 weeks after T cell transfer, progressing to severe colitis after around 6–8 weeks. However, this can vary depending on

the strain used and their microbiota, which will be facility dependent. Although weight loss provides a good method of tracking disease, the onset of severe colitis may be accompanied by a rapid weight loss, which can cause death in a few days. Therefore, once exhibiting signs of disease, mice should be monitored daily and culled before they have lost >20 % of their original weight.

9. The incidence and severity of disease is not always uniform along the entire colon; therefore, samples from different parts should be assessed. Proximal colon samples should be taken from within the first 1–2 cm of the colon; mid colon samples (which often exhibit the most reliable histological changes) taken from the center point; and distal colon samples taken around 1–2 cm from the end of the colon.

10. Plate cultures should be placed into the metal frame inside the anaerobic jar in an upright orientation. Liquid culture flasks should also be securely placed into the metal frame inside the anaerobic jar (use paper towels to wedge flasks into place). To establish a microaerophilic growth environment, close the lid of the anaerobic jar (not too tight or the jar might crack), then attach a vacuum line to one valve and an anaerobic gas cylinder (10 % $CO_2$, 10 % $H_2$, balance $N_2$) to the other. Open the valve to the vacuum and pump out air until the gauge meter on the jar reaches –0.8 bar, then close. Open the valve attached to the anaerobic gas cylinder and fill jar with anaerobic gas mixture until gauge pressure reaches 0 bar, then close. The residual air that was not removed by the vacuum provides enough oxygen to create a microaerophilic atmosphere. Incubate anaerobic jars at 37 °C either standing still (for plates) or on a shaking platform at 150 rpm for liquid cultures. Plate cultures are generally used to start *H. hepaticus* from a frozen aliquot. Incubation for plate culture is 2 days. Following initial plate culture, transfer *H. hepaticus* into liquid culture for subsequent culturing. Liquid cultures need to be split every day. Starting $OD_{600}$ for liquid culture should be 0.05. Note that the *H .hepaticus* liquid cultures do not grow to the same density as most bacterial cultures, rarely exceeding an $OD_{600}$ of 0.5.

11. Note that liquid cultures are much more viable (>90 %) but plate cultures can be used as long as not overgrown (>50 % viable).

## Acknowledgements

K.J.M. is supported by a Wellcome Trust Programme Grant 086354. The authors would like to thank Oliver Harrison, Abhi Kole, Margherita Coccia, and Sofia Nordlander, for help with the preparation of this manuscript.

## References


1. Kaser A, Zeissig S, Blumberg RS (2010) Inflammatory bowel disease. Annu Rev Immunol 28:573
2. Maloy KJ, Powrie F (2011) Intestinal homeostasis and its breakdown in inflammatory bowel disease. Nature 474:298
3. Elson CO et al (2005) Experimental models of inflammatory bowel disease reveal innate, adaptive, and regulatory mechanisms of host dialogue with the microbiota. Immunol Rev 206:260
4. Eckmann L (2006) Animal models of inflammatory bowel disease: lessons from enteric infections. Ann N Y Acad Sci 1072:28
5. Uhlig HH, Powrie F (2009) Mouse models of intestinal inflammation as tools to understand the pathogenesis of inflammatory bowel disease. Eur J Immunol 39:2021
6. Izcue A, Coombes JL, Powrie F (2009) Regulatory lymphocytes and intestinal inflammation. Annu Rev Immunol 27:313
7. Powrie F, Leach MW, Mauze S, Caddle LB, Coffman RL (1993) Phenotypically distinct subsets of CD4+ T cells induce or protect from chronic intestinal inflammation in C. B-17 scid mice. Int Immunol 5:1461
8. Powrie F et al (1994) Inhibition of Th1 responses prevents inflammatory bowel disease in scid mice reconstituted with CD45RBhi CD4+ T cells. Immunity 1:553
9. Powrie F (1995) T cells in inflammatory bowel disease: protective and pathogenic roles. Immunity 3:171
10. Leach MW, Bean AG, Mauze S, Coffman RL, Powrie F (1996) Inflammatory bowel disease in C.B-17 scid mice reconstituted with the CD45RBhigh subset of CD4+ T cells. Am J Pathol 148:1503
11. Bouma G, Strober W (2003) The immunological and genetic basis of inflammatory bowel disease. Nat Rev Immunol 3:521
12. Hue S et al (2006) Interleukin-23 drives innate and T cell-mediated intestinal inflammation. J Exp Med 203:2473
13. Ahern PP et al (2010) Interleukin-23 drives intestinal inflammation through direct activity on T cells. Immunity 33:279
14. Mottet C, Uhlig HH, Powrie F (2003) Cutting edge: cure of colitis by CD4+CD25+ regulatory T cells. J Immunol 170:3939
15. Cahill RJ et al (1997) Inflammatory bowel disease: an immunity-mediated condition triggered by bacterial infection with Helicobacter hepaticus. Infect Immun 65:3126
16. Fox JG, Ge Z, Whary MT, Erdman SE, Horwitz BH (2011) Helicobacter hepaticus infection in mice: models for understanding lower bowel inflammation and cancer. Mucosal Immunol 4:22
17. Kullberg MC et al (2002) Bacteria-triggered CD4(+) T regulatory cells suppress Helicobacter hepaticus-induced colitis. J Exp Med 196:505
18. Kullberg MC et al (2006) IL-23 plays a key role in Helicobacter hepaticus-induced T cell-dependent colitis. J Exp Med 203:2485
19. Jiang HQ, Kushnir N, Thurnheer MC, Bos NA, Cebra JJ (2002) Monoassociation of SCID mice with Helicobacter muridarum, but not four other enterics, provokes IBD upon receipt of T cells. Gastroenterology 122:1346
20. Stepankova R et al (2007) Segmented filamentous bacteria in a defined bacterial cocktail induce intestinal inflammation in SCID mice reconstituted with CD45RBhigh CD4+ T cells. Inflamm Bowel Dis 13:1202
21. Feng S et al (2005) Differential detection of five mouse-infecting helicobacter species by multiplex PCR. Clin Diagn Lab Immunol 12:531
22. Fox JG et al (1998) Hepatic Helicobacter species identified in bile and gallbladder tissue from Chileans with chronic cholecystitis. Gastroenterology 114:755
23. Ge Z, White DA, Whary MT, Fox JG (2001) Fluorogenic PCR-based quantitative detection of a murine pathogen, Helicobacter hepaticus. J Clin Microbiol 39:2598
24. Izcue A et al (2008) Interleukin-23 restrains regulatory T cell activity to drive T cell-dependent colitis. Immunity 28:559
25. Read S, Malmstrom V, Powrie F (2000) Cytotoxic T lymphocyte-associated antigen 4 plays an essential role in the function of CD25(+)CD4(+) regulatory cells that control intestinal inflammation. J Exp Med 192:295
26. Read S et al (2006) Blockade of CTLA-4 on CD4+CD25+ regulatory T cells abrogates their function in vivo. J Immunol 177:4376
27. Morrissey PJ, Charrier K, Braddy S, Liggitt D, Watson JD (1993) CD4+ T cells that express high levels of CD45RB induce wasting disease when transferred into congenic severe combined immunodeficient mice. Disease development is prevented by cotransfer of purified CD4+ T cells. J Exp Med 178:237
28. Maloy KJ et al (2003) CD4+CD25+ T(R) cells suppress innate immune pathology through cytokine dependent mechanisms. J Exp Med 197:111

# Chapter 19

# Analysis of Chromosomal Aberrations in Murine HCC

Kristian Unger and Mathias Heikenwälder

## Abstract

Liver cancer—also called hepatocellular carcinoma (HCC)—is the most frequent primary liver cancer in humans. As of today, it is mainly induced by chronic virus infections such as Hepatitis B and C viruses, which induce chronic hepatitis and fibrosis, the two most important conditions predisposing towards HCC development. Besides, chronic alcohol or drug consumption contributes to chronic liver injury and HCC development. Of note, in industrialized countries virus infections have recently been outcompeted by a high-fat and high-sugar diet as the most important etiology for HCC development in humans—now representing the fastest growing cancer in the USA as of today. It is believed that soon also in Europe high-fat diet caused HCC will become the fastest growing cancer. Today more than 800,000 people die every year due to cancer; however, despite a great research effort in the last 20 years, no efficient curative therapy is available at the moment. It has turned out that various subtypes of HCC exist in humans, complicating the therapy for HCC patients in general, and leading to the need for therapies of stratified patient cohorts as the variability of HCC phenotypes (6 different subtypes exist as of today) influences the responsiveness to treatment. Thus, it is important to dissect and characterize the various HCC subtypes in humans as well as in mouse models to identify the sub-cohorts that are responsive to particular therapies. One step to do so is the characterization of HCC nodules on genetic level. Here, we describe a protocol to characterize individual HCC nodules on genomic level, enabling to stratify the respective liver carcinoma and select them for a more targeted therapy.

**Key words** Hepatocellular carcinoma, HCC, Genomic copy number alterations, FFPE, Array CGH

## 1 Introduction

Today, liver cancer—also called hepatocellular carcinoma (HCC)—reflects the third most common cause for cancer related death worldwide with approximately 800,000 deaths per year. In stray African or Asian countries HCC has become the most common cause for cancer-related death, mainly as a consequence of viral infections with Hepatitis B and C viruses (HBV; HCV). As of today 550 million people are persistently infected with HBV or HCV. In addition, chronic or acute intoxication (e.g., alcohol, drug abuse, aflatoxin-b) is a known risk factor to cause HCC, but responsible only for a relatively small number of cases.

Ari Waisman and Burkhard Becher (eds.), *T-Helper Cells: Methods and Protocols*, Methods in Molecular Biology, vol. 1193, DOI 10.1007/978-1-4939-1212-4_19, 

In addition to accumulating patient numbers with HBV or HCV induced HCC, which for sure represents a clinical health problem, our lifestyle has become a major factor driving inflammatory liver disease—thereby strongly increasing the risk to develop liver cancer. A combination of high-fat, high-sugar diet and little exercise additionally worsens this problematic development. Indeed, it was shown that dietary and genetic obesity promotes non-alcoholic steatohepatitis (NASH); (pathologic hepatic lipid deposition and hepatitis) and tumorigenesis. Notably, in Europe and the USA the prevalence of HCC is strongly increasing, reflecting the fastest increasing cancer type in the USA, and prospectively this trend will worsen further.

Given the effort that has been invested in the past to understand and treat HCC—induced by viruses, high-fat diet, or chronic alcohol consumption—clinical success has been extremely small. Various novel drugs have been investigated. Although these regimens are successful approaches to prolong the life span of liver cancer patients—these drugs are rather palliative than curative. Up to now liver transplantation has been the most effective way to prolong the life span of patients—but in 50 % of the cases cancer comes back.

Importantly, HCC does not resemble a single entity but rather a diverse spectrum of cancers in humans. In many cases individual patients carry different liver cancer subtypes, distinct not only in their morphology, their genetics and epigenetics but also in their composition of inflammatory cells. Personalized therapeutic approaches will be needed in future—depending on the tumor type, the tumor stage as well as the individual composition of distinct liver cancers in one and the same patient. Due to the above outlined problems a systemic, therapeutic approach to treat liver cancer in humans is not available—underlining the urgent need for new targets that can be included in basic research and clinical trials. In the light of the above modeling, liver cancer in rodents appears to be very important, but the kind of human pathology resembled by a mouse model and the degree of clinical success in preclinical models that can be translated to a human HCC subtype need to be analysed. Thus, a stratification of HCC in mice and human is needed to identify the respective HCC subtypes and—hopefully—the individual efficient therapies for the stratified patient cohorts. To do so one aim is to analyze chromosomal aberrations of individual HCC—in order to define, subtype, and characterize HCC.

## 2 Materials

- Qiagen QIAmp DNA Microkit (QIAGEN).
- NanoDrop spectrophotometer (Thermo).
- Qubit fluorometer (Invitrogen).

- Agilent hybridization oven (Agilent).
- Agilent Microarray Scanner (Agilent).
- 1 M Sodium thiocyanate (NaSCN).
- Amicon 30 kDa filter columns (Millipore).
- Enzo oligo array CGH labeling kit (Enzo).
- DNA Suspension Buffer (Teknova).
- QIAmp DNA Microkit (Qiagen).
- Xylene.
- Ethanol abs., 90 and 70 %.
- Multiplex PCR primers with sequences as described in Van Beers et al. [1].
- High-quality PCR kit such as the FastStart High Fidelity PCR System (Roche).
- Paraformaldehyde (4 %) for fixation.
- Dehydration and paraffin embedding machine to generate paraffin blocks.

## 3 Methods

### 3.1 Mouse Tissue Formalin Fixation, Paraffin Embedding, and Preparation of Samples

We first generate formalin-fixed paraffin-embedded blocks (FFPE; 4 % PFA fixed) of livers with macroscopic tumor nodules and cut consecutive sections, each 2 μm thick. To do so the following steps should be performed:

- After removing the liver take the liver lobe that macroscopically contains a tumor nodule (*see* Fig. 1).
  - Shortly rinse tissue after dissection with sterile isotonic NaCl (0.9 %) or PBS to get rid of blood.
  - Put tissue for FFPE in 4 % PFA (at least five times of tissue weight; make sure that PFA is clear during fixation—otherwise change PFA once) and incubate for at least 48 h at room temperature (or 72–96 h at 4 °C). Fixation depends on size and consistency of tissue. (i.e., consider pre-cutting or longer fixation for large/stroma enriched tumors)
  - If you desire special nuclear staining, fixation in PFA has to be prolonged up to 5 days at room temperature. This can also be achieved by fixing a precut section before staining, consequently not over-fixing the whole tissue.
  - In case of longer storage of tissue before alcohol dehydration and paraffin embedding you might store fixed tissue in sterile PBS at 4 °C for up to 1 week maximum.
  - If prefixed, non-embedded tissue is to be sent at room temperature, please consider putting the fixed tissue in

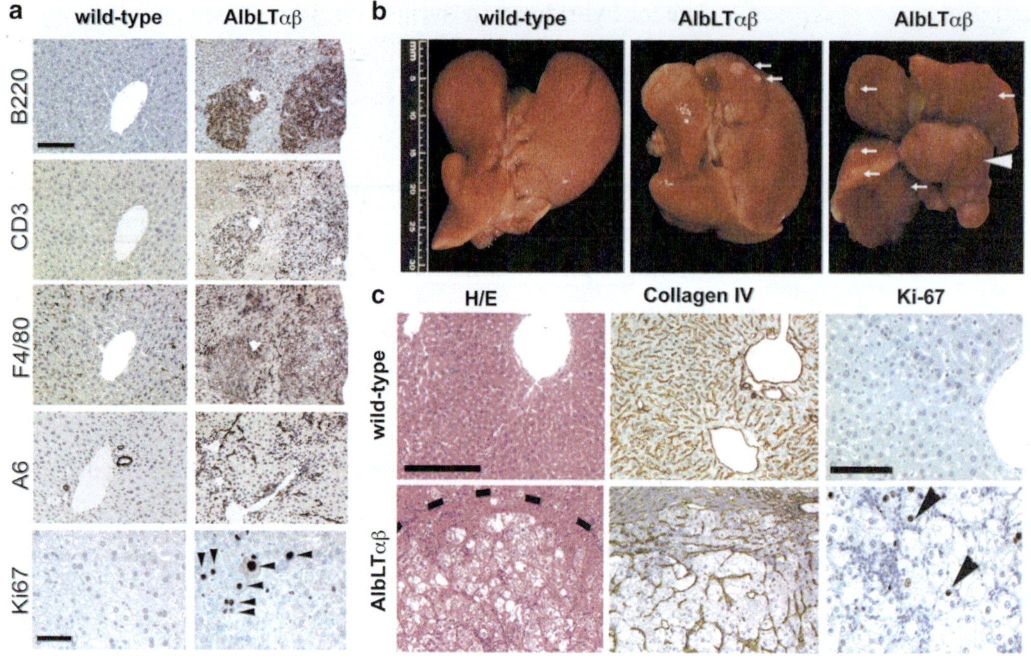


**Fig. 1** Chronic inflammation-induced liver damage and HCC in AlbLTαβ mice. (**a**) Immunohistochemistry of representative livers from 9-month-old C57BL/6 and AlbLTαβ mice. B220+ B cells, CD3+ T cells, F4/80+ macrophages, Kupffer cells (scale bar: 150 μm). Ki67+, proliferating hepatocytes (*arrowheads*), or inflammatory cells are indicated (scale bar: 50 μm). (**b**, *left two panels*) Macroscopy of C57BL/6 and AlbLTαβ livers. *White arrows* indicate tumor nodules. *White arrowhead* indicates a complete liver lobe affected by HCC. (**b**, *right four panels*) Liver histology of 12-month-old C57BL/6 and AlbLTαβ mice. Collagen IV staining highlights the broadening of the liver cell cords; loss of collagen IV networks indicates HCC (scale bar: 200 μm). High numbers of Ki67+ proliferating hepatocytes (*arrowheads*) in AlbLTαβ HCC (scale bar: 100 μm). (**c**) Immunohistochemical analysis of a clear cell HCC, that display broadening of the Collagen IV positive liver plates as well as proliferating Ki67 positive hepatocytes (H and E; KI67 and Collagen IV). Adapted from [1]

0.4–1 % PFA—diluted with PBS (always use isotonic solutions and make sure that flask is completely filled).

- Cutting tissue prior to alcohol dehydration and paraffin embedding: Always use the same liver lobes and cut in the same direction. If you have more than one lobe, you might consider cutting one horizontally (axial/transversal) to big vessels and the other sagittal in 5 mm thick sections. Further, paraffin blocks are cut and 2 μm thick sections are put on glass slides in order to prepare them for histological and immune-histological staining.

The sections are stained on a BOND-MAX staining roboter from Leica for Collagen IV, Ki67, GOLPH2, glutamine synthetase, β-Catenin, and H/E (Fig. 1). Based on these results the regions that reflect HCC can be defined (between 0.5 and 20 mm in diameter) and those regions can be stabbed out—presumably HCC—out of the paraffin block [2] for further genomic analyses.

### 3.2 Isolation and Quality Control of Genomic DNA from FFPE Tissue Cylinders

- The tissue cylinders are deparaffinized three times in xylene at room temperature and then washed in absolute, 96 %, and 70 % ethanol for 30 s each.
- The tissue is allowed to dry briefly, to allow the ethanol to evaporate; the tissue is moistened with nuclease-free water and transferred into a 1.5 ml eppendorf, then air-dried for 10–15 min
- One milliliter of 1 M sodium thiocyanate (NaSCN) is added to the eppendorf, vortexed, and then incubated overnight at 38 °C to breakdown DNA cross-links.
- The following day, the sample is centrifuged, the supernatant removed, and then washed twice with PBS to remove the NaSCN.
- The DNA extraction then follows the Qiagen QIAmp DNA Microkit (QIAGEN) standard protocol: addition of 60 μl ATL buffer, and 60 μl proteinase K, and incubation at 55 °C until the tissue is digested
- Incubation at 98 °C for 10 min; 100 μl ATL buffer is added, then 200 μl AL buffer; the sample gets vortexed, then 200 μl ethanol is added and incubated at room temperature for 5 min.
- The lysate is transferred to the QIAamp MinElute Column (300 μl each time) and spun at 6,800 × *g* for 1 min (300 μl of sample is added and spun down until all the sample gets transferred to the column).
- 500 μl AW1 buffer is added and spun at 6,800 × *g* for 1 min.
- 500 μl AW2 buffer is added and spun for 1 min at 6,800 × *g*, and 3 min at full speed to dry the membrane.
- 30 μl of AE buffer (depending on initial sample tissue size) is added to the column to elute the DNA followed by incubation for 5 min and then spun at 6,800 × *g* into a clean eppendorf to collect the DNA sample.
- The sample is then quantified using the NanoDrop spectrophotometer (ND-2000), blanked with AE buffer
- In order to obtain the exact DNA concentration, the sample is quantified using the Qubit fluorophotometer
- The DNA is subsequently stored at 4 °C for up to a year and for longer-term storage at −20 °C

### 3.3 DNA Quality Integrity Check by Multiplex-PCR

A gene-specific multiplex PCR [1] is used with PCR primers for the housekeeping gene GDP resulting in 100 bp-, 200 bp-, 300 bp-, and 400 bp non-overlapping amplicons, respectively. Only samples with an amplifiable fragment size of greater than 200 bp are suitable for further processing by array CGH.

### 3.4 Array CGH

A critical decision that has to be taken is the proper selection of the appropriate array platform that mainly depends on the type and quality of the starting material. Oligo array CGH arrays from Agilent with 60mer oligonucleotide probes have been proven to work very well with suboptimal quality DNA resulting from formalin-induced degradation in FFPE tissues [3]. Further, the workflow we use for array CGH analysis includes labeling of DNA using the "CGH labeling kit for oligo arrays" from Enzo. Compared to other kits, in our hands, this kit results in much better incorporation efficiencies and better array CGH profiles when using degraded DNA from FFPE samples. The incorporation efficiency of Cy3 or Cy5 is determined by the so-called "specific activity," which is the incorporation of labeled nucleotides normalized by the overall concentration of DNA in the labeled sample. Recommendations for optimal specific activities are given in the Agilent array CGH protocol; however, in our experience there is no fixed threshold predicting success of the experiment. When carrying out hybridization of the labeled samples, we split the experiment in batches of reasonable size (max. five slides per batch) and start with those samples with the highest specific activities. As the specific activities decrease with higher batches, the success of hybridization, visible by the resulting array CGH profiles, drops off at some point. We do not hybridize samples with a specific activity lower than that of the last successful batch.

#### 3.4.1 Array CGH Labeling

The Enzo CGH Labeling Kit for Oligo Arrays is used for labeling. Firstly the DNA is denatured, and random primers annealed. For this the following components are added to a 1.5 ml eppendorf:

- Water 19—$x$µl.
- Primers/Reaction buffer—20 µl.
- DNA—$x$µl (500 ng, max 19 µl).
- Total volume—39 µl.
- The contents are then heated at 99 °C for 10 min and placed on ice for 2 min.

The primers are extended using Klenow Exo-DNA Polymerase by adding the following components:

- To test sample, 10 µl Cy3.
- To reference sample, 10 µl Cy5.
- Klenow Exo-DNA Polymerase to both (Cy3 and Cy5) samples: 1 µl.
- The contents are then incubated at 37 °C for 4 h and the reaction stopped with 5 µl of Stop Buffer.
- Cleanup/purification of the labeled DNA is performed using Amicon 30 kDa filter columns.

- 430 μl of DNA suspension buffer is added to each reaction tube, then the sample is added to the Amicon 30 kDa filter column, and spun for 10 min at 14,000 × *g* at room temperature.
- The sample is further purified by adding 480 μl of DNA suspension buffer and spinning for 10 min.
- The sample is recovered by inverting the filter into a fresh 1.5-mL eppendorf and spinning for 1 min at 1,000 × *g* at room temperature.
- The required volume of the purified sample is 39 μl.

The NanoDrop is used to measure the yield and specific activity using 1.5 μl of sample and the following calculations:

$$\text{Yield}(\mu g) = \text{DNA concentration}(ng/\mu l) \times \text{Sample volume } (\mu l) / 1{,}000 \text{ } ng/\mu g$$

$$\text{Specific activity} = \text{pmol per l dye} / \mu g \text{ per } \mu l \text{ genomic DNA}$$

According to the Array-based CGH for Genomic DNA Analysis Protocol (Agilent), acceptable values for hybridization of labeled DNA were: a yield of 5–7 μg and specific activity of Cy3 of 25–40 pmol/μg and a specific activity of Cy5 of 20–35 pmol/μg.

#### 3.4.2 Array CGH Hybridization, Washing, and Scanning

For hybridization the Cy5 and Cy3-labeled samples are combined and the following components added:

- 5 μl Cot-1 DNA (1.0 mg/mL).
- 11 μl Agilent 10× Blocking Agent.
- 55 μl Agilent 2× Hi-RPM Buffer.
- 71 μl Hybridization Master Mix.
- The sample is incubated at 95 °C for 3 min and then immediately transferred to a heat block at 37 °C for 30 min for prehybridization (hybridization of cot-1 DNA with repetitive sequences of labeled DNA).
- The sample is then applied to a gasket slide.
- The active side of the microarray is placed on top of the gasket slide to form a "sandwich slide pair," the chamber closed, and transferred to the hybridization oven (Agilent) and rotated at 65 °C for 24 h at a rotational speed of 20 rpm.

Washing and scanning of slides is performed as per Agilent protocol, using Oligo aCGH Wash Buffer 1 and 2. Slides are washed at room temperature with Agilent Oligo aCGH Wash Buffer 1 for 5 min and with Agilent Oligo aCGH Wash Buffer 2 for 1 min at 37 °C, then air-dried.

Array slides are scanned using a microarray scanner with 3 μm resolution (Agilent), which generates a two-layer tiff file with one image of Cy3 and one of Cy5 fluorescence.

It is very important that hybridization and washing that involve some steps such as assembly and disassembly of the hybridization "sandwich," which require some practice, are carried out or supervised by staff with experience in this technique. Also, particular care has to be taken when it comes to adjusting and controlling the temperatures during the hybridization and washing procedures. For the sake of reproducibility, it is extremely important that an experiment is carried out by only the same person in order to make sure that all steps are done the same way.

Since ozone which degrades Cy5 and thereby the overall signal of the reference channel can be a problem, particularly on hot summer days, we highly recommend to filter the air of the microarray lab with an activated carbon filter.

#### 3.4.3 Extraction of Fluorescence Intensities, Data Analysis, and Visualization

The scanned images (two-layer tiff files) are further processed with the Feature Extraction Software (Agilent), which writes the measured fluorescence intensities into text files and also generates a quality report for each of the processed scanned image files. The quality report comes with the three quality categories "excellent," "good," and "evaluate" whilst the latter indicates problems with the data. However, it has to be noted that the thresholds for these categories were defined for non-degraded DNA of optimal quality and do not apply for DNA from FFPE samples. Therefore, negative quality reports do not necessarily mean that the data are not useful in downstream analysis.

With regard to data analysis, we use a workflow that is specifically tailored for tissue sample analysis and FFPE tissue samples in particular [4]. It takes into account the fact that the resulting data which basically reflect the fluorescence intensities from the Cy3 channel (normally sample DNA) and the Cy5 channel (normally reference DNA), respectively, are more noisy compared to that from fresh tissue samples or cultured cells. This noise is mainly caused by a fraction of very small DNA fragments that unspecifically hybridize in a random manner to the microarray probes. Since it is impossible to get rid of this experimental noise, one has to deal with it in downstream data analysis. This consists of the following steps: data import, quality filtering, normalization, segmentation, copy number calling, complexity reduction, and statistical testing. We do all this within the R statistical platform [5] on a Linux server in combination with functions from the Bioconductor packages CGHcall [6] and CGHregions [7] and in-house written functions.

After importing the data by reading in the text files, the data, data points not fulfilling our quality criteria are excluded from further analysis. Beside others the most important criteria are replicate consistency and foreground-to-background ratio. If the deviation between replicates is too high, i.e., >10 %, the appropriate data points are excluded. For the foreground-to-background ratio we apply a threshold of 2.5, i.e., the foreground signal of a data point has to be 2.5 times the local background signal. In data filtering the majority of excluded data points are excluded because of a suboptimal foreground-to-background ratio. Before applying normalization, which in our case is simple median normalization, we correct the ratios for local (spatial) differences in the hybridization patterns. We frequently observe that the overall hybridization signal slightly differs across the slide. These artifacts can heavily bias the results and are the result of uncontrollable effects caused by handling of the slides during hybridization and washing. In order to control for these artifacts, we apply the MANOR [8] method (Fig. 3) which calculates an average signal for each locus on the slide using LOESS regression and uses the resulting coefficient for correction. The corrected ratios are log2-transformed and median-normalized before subjected to segmentation and calling of the copy number. The segmentation algorithm [9] uses the data points that are ordered according to their genomic position and divides them into segments of the same copy number whilst there is one median ratio for each of the segments. In the next step the copy number segments are called according to their underlying copy number. This step highly depends on the cellularity, i.e., the proportion of tumor cells in the analyzed tissue sample and the used CGHcall algorithm [6] takes this into account. This allows to accurately type the copy numbers and to include the assessment of the tumor cell cellularity. Each segment then is assigned a copy number in the form double-loss, single-loss, normal, gain, high-level amplification, the latter resembling a copy number of greater than five.

Detailed Description of Raw-Data Import, Preprocessing, Segmentation, and Copy Number Calling

- In the first step we read in complete text files as generated by the Agilent Feature Extraction software and skip the first 9 lines since these only contain meta-information that is not used in further analysis.
- From the imported data we only keep the columns that we need for further analysis which are as follows:
  - Col, Row, GeneName, SystematicName, ProbeName: metainformation of the positions of the probes on the array and probe IDs.
  - rMedianSignal and gMedianSignal: foreground median signals of the “red” Cy5 and the “green” Cy3 channels.
  - rBGMedianSignal and gBGMedianSignal: background median signals of the Cy5 and Cy3 channels.
  - ControlType: information on whether a probe is control—only non-controls are kept in the analysis.
- The resulting reduced data matrices are then subjected to spatial normalization using the MANOR [8] method. In order to see the R code that is used for this step, please refer to

the MANOR documentation (http://www.bioconductor.org/packages/release/bioc/html/MANOR.html). The method also excludes technical outlier data points.

- After median normalization and background correction (background signal subtracted from the foreground signal of each channel applied) on the spatially corrected data, the built log2 ratios are collected in a new data matrix that contains the following columns:
  - Name (Agilent array probe name), Chromosome (chromosome the probe relates to), Start (probe start position on the chromosome in bp), End (probe end position on the chromosome in bp).
  - The following columns contain the normalized log2 ratios from each array to be analyzed.
- The normalized data matrix is then subjected to preprocessing, segmentation, copy number calling, and the definition of copy number regions.
- For copy number calling we apply the function CGHcall from the CGHcall [6] package. In order to make the function work most accurately we need to provide the cellularity (i.e., the proportion of tumor cells in the whole sample analyzed). The cellularity needs to be assessed from H and E stained FFPE sections of the tissue to be analyzed. Alternatively, if no cellularities are available gross estimates (e.g., 80 %) can be used.
- The R code applied for these steps is very well documented in the manuals of the CGHcall [6] and CGHregions [7] packages (http://www.bioconductor.org/packages/release/bioc/vignettes/ CGHcall/inst/doc/CGHcall.pdf, http://www.bioconductor.org/packages/release/bioc/html/CGHregions.html). Also an example script resembling all described steps of analysis can be downloaded at http://www.helmholtz-muenchen.de/zyto/research/groups/integrative-biology/software/index.html.

Before association analysis the copy number called data need to be reduced in complexity, i.e., the number of tests. Without this reduction one ends up with hundreds of segments to be tested for association with any parameters (e.g., knockdown vs. control) and such a high number of tests comes with the so-called multiple testing problem. This means that with a $p$-value threshold $\alpha$ of 0.05 one would expect 5 % false-positive results. Since this is not acceptable, one has to control for this by $p$-value adjustment. The extent of this adjustment correlates with the total number of tests, so reduction of data complexity increases the statistical power of the approach. The complexity of array CGH data can be reduced by summarizing segments in a sequence and of the same copy number to copy number regions which is done by the CGHregions [7] method. Applying this allows to reduce the number of tests from usually greater 1,000 to around 100–200 tests. The *p*-values resulting from simple *t*-testing are then corrected using the Benjamini–Hochberg method [10].

- In order to test for associations of copy number with any parameter, a text file needs to be generated containing the information on the parameters (columns) to be tested for each of the samples included in the study (lines). The order of samples (lines) in the text file has to be same as in the CGHregions object.
- The text file is read into R and stored as a data frame object with the name "dataclinvar".
- Testing is performed using the CGHtest R package (http://www.few.vu.nl/~mavdwiel/CGHtest.html) which has to be installed and loaded.
- The CGHtest method uses the copy number calls from the CGHregions object in combination with the dataclinvar object in order to calculate the frequencies of each state (−2 total loss, −1 single loss, 0 normal, 1 gain, 2 high-level amplification) in the groups to be defined by the parameter (e.g., treated vs. non-treated). The group-wise frequencies are calculated for each state separately and then subjected to testing. In order to define which variable has to be tested one has to give the number of the appropriate parameter of the dataclinvar table. The testing can then be performed whilst the user can choose between different test-statistics (by default chi-square testing is used).
- The resulting table contains the genomic location and size of the copy number region to be tested, the group-wise frequencies and the *p*-value.
- In a next step the *p*-values are corrected for multiple-testing error and the false-discovery rate FDR is estimated by permutation. This step is computationally intensive and if possible the parallel-computing option should be chosen that allows using all processors available on the computer or server to be used.
- This finally results in a table containing the data from the results table before complemented by a column with the FDR values. The table is written into a text or Excel file for assessment of statistically significant copy number changes.

Further, the results can be visualized in karyogram-like plots in order to see group-specific chromosomal copy number alterations or subjected to unsupervised cluster analysis that groups similar copy number profiles and thereby allows to test possible associations of global copy number changes with any biological parameter.

For karyogram-like plots (Fig. 2) an in-house written R function (http://www.helmholtz-muenchen.de/zyto/research/groups/integrative-biology/software/index.html) is used. This function accepts either CGHcall or CGHregions objects and plots the copy

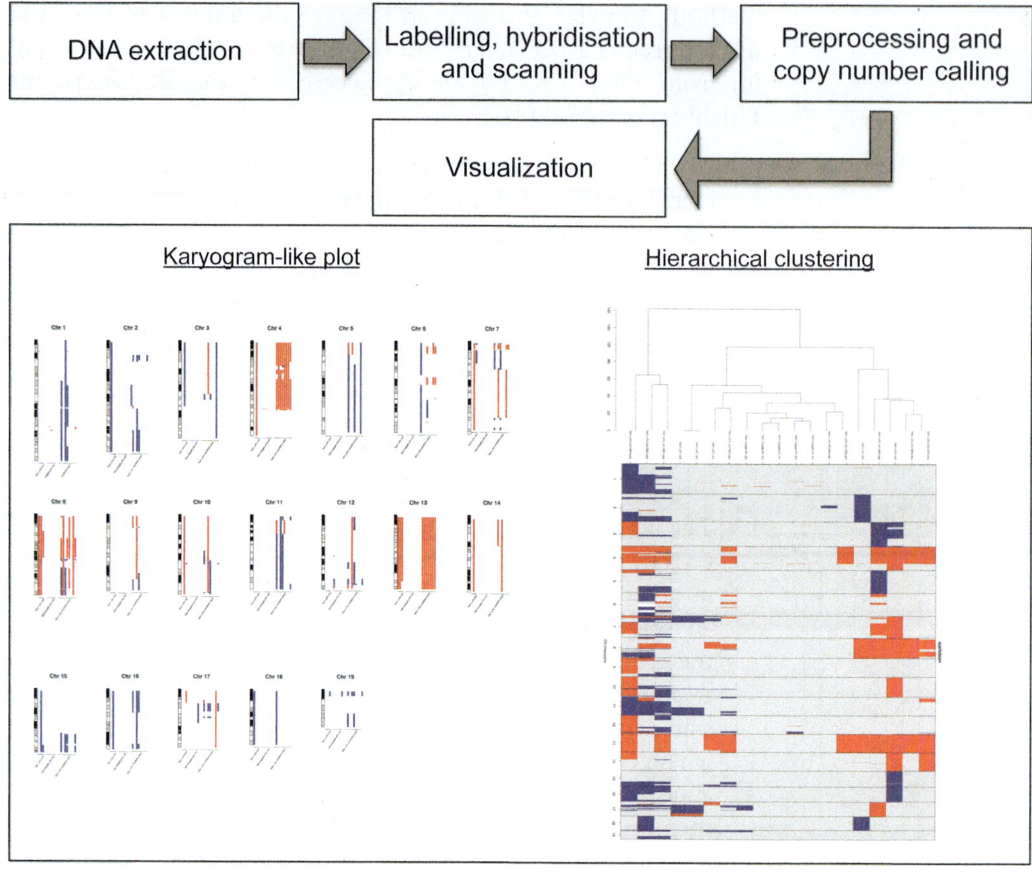


**Fig. 2** Workflow of the analysis on chromosomal aberrations in murine HCC. FFPE tailored extraction of genomic DNA from tissue cylinders is followed by fluorescence labeling of sample and reference DNA and subsequent hybridization onto high-resolution oligo array CGH arrays. The fluorescence intensities are extracted from the images and subjected to data preprocessing including spatial normalization. Finally the copy number status for all copy number probes is calculated and the resulting array CGH profiles plotted according to their genomic positions (*bottom left*: karyogram-like plot) or in form of a heatmap while the profiles are sorted according to similarity of copy number patterns (*red*: copy number gain, *blue*: copy number loss). The raw-data relating to a study by Reisinger et al. [11] were downloaded from ArrayExpress (http://www.ebi.ac.uk/arrayexpress; accession number E-MTAB-1559)

number changes chromosome-by-chromosome according to their chromosomal positions. The function allows to select specific colors used for drawing gain and lost copy number regions.

For drawing heatmaps of the copy number calls or copy number regions according to hierarchical clustering (Fig. 2) also an inhouse written R function (http://www.helmholtz-muenchen.de/zyto/research/groups/integrative-biology/software/index.html) is used that only requires the CGHcall or CGHregions object in order to work. The function allows to select the parameters for clustering (distance and linkage methods) and also the colors used in the plot (Fig. 3).

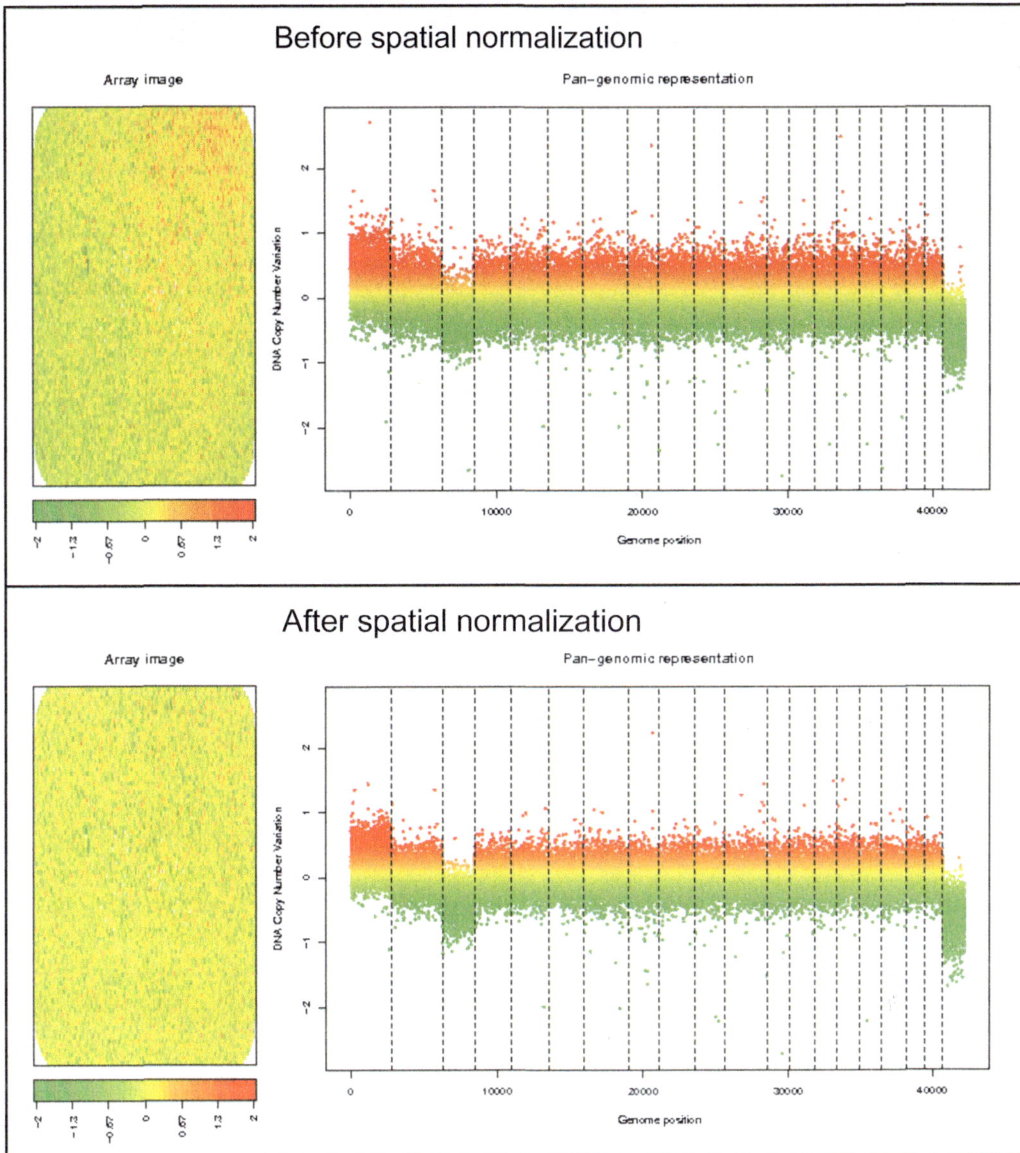


**Fig. 3** Spatial normalization for the correction of hybridization artifacts. In the *upper panel* a nonuniform hybridization pattern is visible with a trend of higher log2-ratio intensities in the *upper-right corner* of the array and lower log2 intensities in the *lower-bottom corner*. Uniformity of hybridization is recovered after MANOR normalization

## References


1. Haybaeck J et al (2009) A lymphotoxin-driven pathway to hepatocellular carcinoma. Cancer Cell 16:295–308
2. Van Beers EH et al (2006) A multiplex PCR predictor for aCGH success of FFPE samples. Br J Cancer 94:333–337
3. Hess J et al (2011) Gain of chromosome band 7q11 in papillary thyroid carcinomas of young patients is associated with exposure to low-dose irradiation. Proc Natl Acad Sci U S A 108: 9595–9600
4. Zitzelsberger H, Unger K (2011) DNA copy number alterations in radiation-induced thyroid cancer. Clin Oncol 23:289–296
5. R Core Team (2013) R: a language and environment for statistical computing. R Foundation

for Statistical Computing. http://www.R-project.org

6. Van de Wiel MA et al (2007) CGHcall: calling aberrations for array CGH tumor profiles. Bioinformatics 23:892–894
7. Van de Wiel MA, van Wieringen WN (2007) CGHregions: dimension reduction for array CGH data with minimal information loss. Cancer Inform 3:55–63
8. Neuvial P et al (2006) Spatial normalization of array-CGH data. BMC Bioinformatics 7: 264
9. Venkatraman ES, Olshen AB (2007) A faster circular binary segmentation algorithm for the analysis of array CGH data. Bioinformatics 23:657–663
10. Benjamini Y, Yekutieli D (2005) Quantitative trait loci analysis using the false discovery rate. Genetics 171:783–790
11. Vucur M et al (2013) RIP3 inhibits inflammatory hepatocarcinogenesis but promotes cholestasis by controlling caspase-8- and JNK-dependent compensatory cell proliferation. Cell Rep 4:776–790

# Index



Ari Waisman and Burkhard Becher (eds.), *T-Helper Cells: Methods and Protocols*, Methods in Molecular Biology, vol. 1193, DOI 10.1007/978-1-4939-1212-4, © Springer Science+Business Media New York 2014

9781493912117